T0001514

The Essential
Guide to Adaptogens

The Essential Guide to Adaptogens

15 SUPER HERBS TO RELIEVE COMMON AILMENTS

Dr. Rachel Rozelle

ROCKRIDGE PRESS

Copyright © 2020 by Rockridge Press, Emeryville, California

No part of this publication may be reproduced, stored in a retrieval system, or transmitted in any form or by any means, electronic, mechanical, photocopying, recording, scanning, or otherwise, except as permitted under Sections 107 or 108 of the 1976 United States Copyright Act, without the prior written permission of the Publisher. Requests to the Publisher for permission should be addressed to the Permissions Department, Rockridge Press, 6005 Shellmound Street, Suite 175, Emeryville, CA 94608.

Limit of Liability/Disclaimer of Warranty: The Publisher and the author make no representations or warranties with respect to the accuracy or completeness of the contents of this work and specifically disclaim all warranties, including without limitation warranties of fitness for a particular purpose. No warranty may be created or extended by sales or promotional materials. The advice and strategies contained herein may not be suitable for every situation. This work is sold with the understanding that the Publisher is not engaged in rendering medical, legal, or other professional advice or services. If professional assistance is required, the services of a competent professional person should be sought. Neither the Publisher nor the author shall be liable for damages arising herefrom. The fact that an individual, organization, or website is referred to in this work as a citation and/or potential source of further information does not mean that the author or the Publisher endorses the information the individual, organization, or website may provide or recommendations they/it may make. Further, readers should be aware that websites listed in this work may have changed or disappeared between when this work was written and when it is read.

For general information on our other products and services or to obtain technical support, please contact our Customer Care Department within the United States at (866) 744-2665, or outside the United States at (510) 253-0500.

Rockridge Press publishes its books in a variety of electronic and print formats. Some content that appears in print may not be available in electronic books, and vice versa.

TRADEMARKS: Rockridge Press and the Rockridge Press logo are trademarks or registered trademarks of Callisto Media Inc. and/or its affiliates, in the United States and other countries, and may not be used without written permission. All other trademarks are the property of their respective owners. Rockridge Press is not associated with any product or vendor mentioned in this book.

Interior and Cover Designer: Carlos Esparza
Art Producer: Janice Ackerman
Editor: Nicky Montalvo
Production Editor: Rachel Taenzler

Cover Photography: Courtesy of Shutterstock. Interior Photography: Courtesy of Shutterstock; vi: Courtesy of istock. Author photo: Courtesy of Melanie Roberts.

ISBN: Print 978-1-64739-903-0 | eBook 978-1-64739-904-7
R0

I dedicate this book to my loving family, who have always supported me, and continue to support me in all of my endeavors.

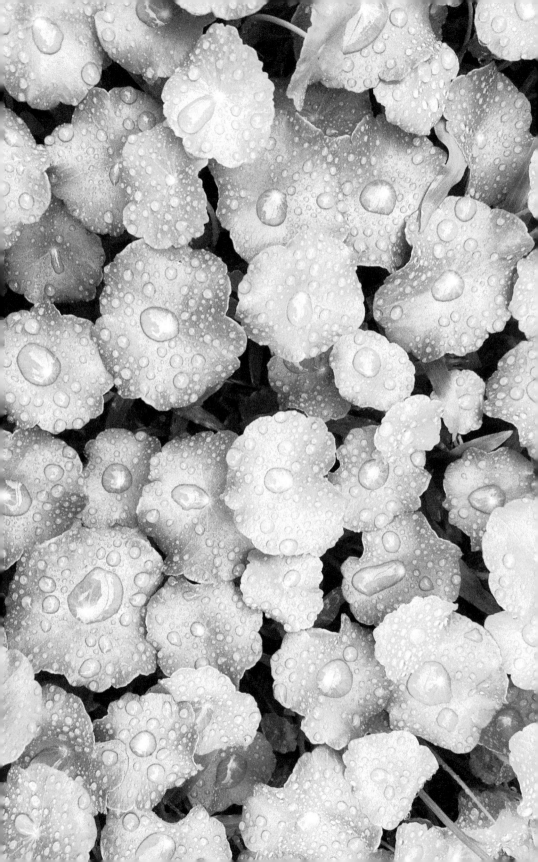

Contents

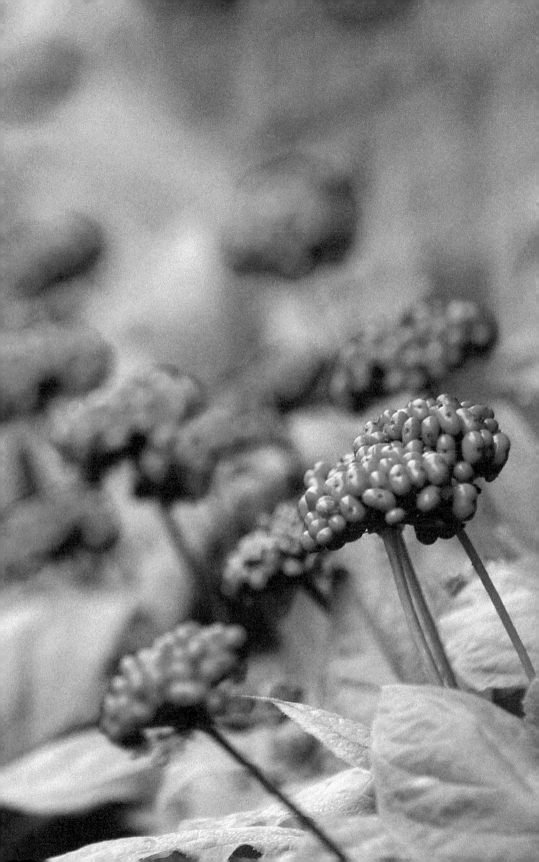

Introduction

My love for botanical medicine started when I was in medical school and has only grown from there. The more I have used herbs, the more awed I have been by their range of usefulness and the beauty of their healing abilities.

As a naturopathic doctor, I frequently hear unfortunate stories from patients who haven't been supported by conventional medicine. These stories break my heart. Whether it's being told that there are no treatment options, that a lifetime of pharmaceuticals is the only answer, or that herbs and supplements don't work (by medical doctors who haven't been trained in or looked deeply at plant-based medicine), patients are left feeling discouraged, defeated, powerless, and without options. I hope this book can help change that paradigm of medical thinking and serve as a testament that there are many safe and effective natural treatment options for various conditions.

Vis medicatrix naturae means "the healing power of nature" and is a foundational concept within naturopathic medicine. Naturopathic doctors believe our bodies have incredible healing abilities, and that plant-based medicine works powerfully with the body to promote that healing. My biggest goals with this book are to increase awareness of natural treatment options and help educate and empower readers to be their own health-care advocates.

Unlike conventional medications, medicinal plants and fungi perform multiple therapeutic actions on the body. Most botanical medicines are much safer than pharmaceuticals, featuring far fewer side effects, and can also be specially formulated to each individual. There are many different classifications of botanicals based upon their actions. Among all of them, I believe the adaptogens are the most important.

Adaptogens can be thought of as "herbal armor" because of their ability to protect our bodies from various modern stressors, including emotional stress, environmental toxins, and infectious diseases. Supporting the detoxification pathways, immune system, hormone system, nervous system, and more, adaptogens help the body manage and recover from a range of challenges.

In my clinical practice, I have used adaptogenic herbs more than any other type of herb because of their wide range of physiological effects on the body and their ability to modulate the stress response. Excessive stress is a common "obstacle to cure" in my patients. Removing those stressors and modulating that stress response has been essential to their healing.

Adaptogenic herbs, when used correctly alongside a healthy diet and lifestyle, can support your vitality, resilience, and innate healing mechanisms.

This book is your ultimate resource on how to use adaptogens to heal, invigorate, and stress-proof your mind and body.

Note: This book offers guidelines to the consumer on how to effectively use adaptogens to support their health. The information in this book is not intended to replace medical care from a physician.

How to Use This Book

It is recommended to read this book in its entirety from beginning to end. As tempting as it is to just dive in and start using these miraculous herbs, to get the most value out of their use, it is important to first gain a fundamental understanding of what adaptogens are and how they work in the body. This book will give you foundational knowledge about adaptogens and their history and then guide you to use them yourself to restore balance and resilience to your body.

We will discuss each adaptogen in detail, as each one has unique healing properties and many work most effectively when consumed with other remedies. Understanding these differences will help you determine which adaptogens may be of most benefit to you personally and how to effectively use them to achieve and maintain your own health goals.

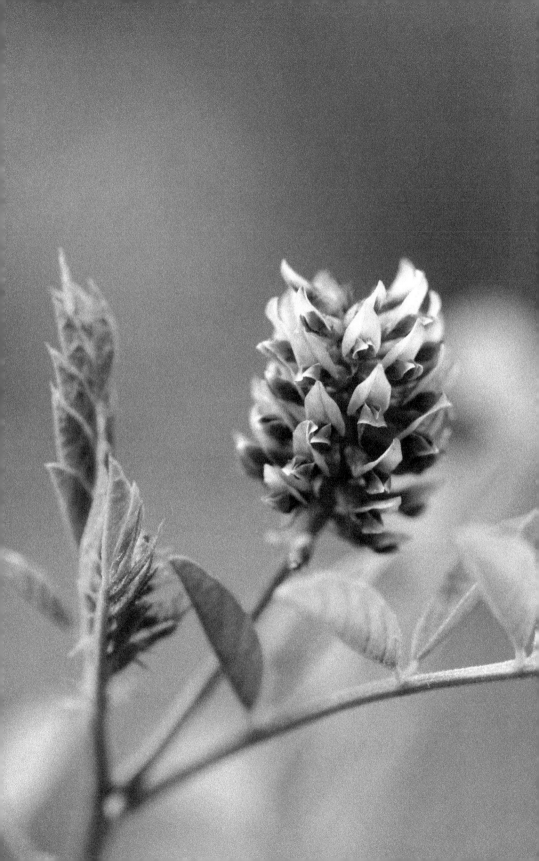

PART ONE

Understand

Before we profile each adaptogen, we will lay the groundwork of what an adaptogen is by discussing in great detail what qualities make a plant an adaptogen and how this definition originally came about. We will explore some of the first spiritual, mythical, and medicinal uses of these plants and fungi, as well as how they are used today.

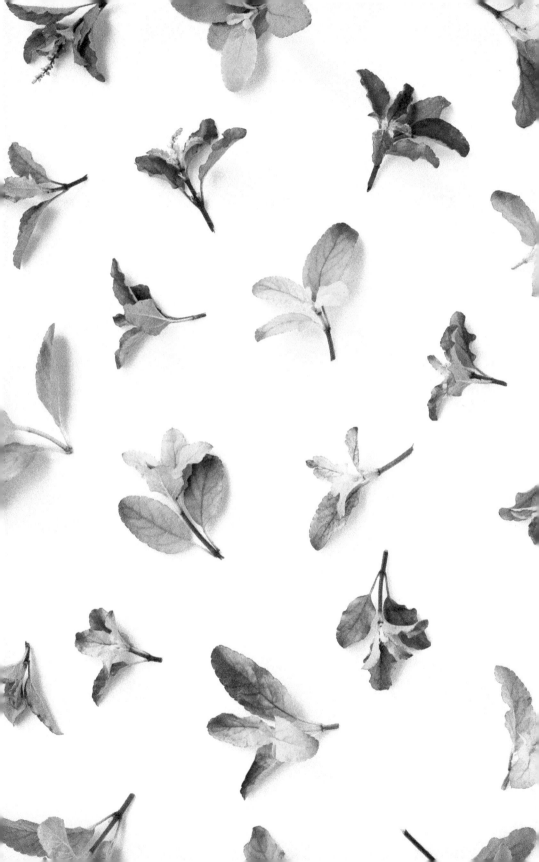

CHAPTER ONE

Adaptogens: Why We Love Them

There are many reasons to love adaptogens. Adaptogens are remarkable plants and fungi that have numerous therapeutic effects on the body and mind. They provide benefits for immune health, sleep, hormone balance, brain function, energy, and so much more! In this chapter, we will explain what makes adaptogens special and explore the fascinating history of how and why they were discovered. These medicinal plants and fungi have been used for thousands of years due to their remarkable healing abilities. Their resilience and ability to survive in harsh and changing climates over centuries speak volumes about their ability to adapt to and withstand stress.

Adaptogens Defined

Although adaptogens have been used for thousands of years, the scientific term "adaptogen" was not officially defined or found in scientific literature until the 1900s.

The term *adaptogen* was officially coined in 1957 by Dr. Nikolai Lazarev. Dr. Lazarev defined adaptogens as substances that increase the state of nonspecific resistance to stress. In 1968, his colleagues Dr. Israel I. Brekhman and Dr. I. V. Dardymov expanded upon this definition, characterizing adaptogens as substances that:

- are nontoxic to the body's physiological functions
- produce a nonspecific state of resistance to various stressors, including physiological, chemical, and biological traumas
- must have an overall normalizing effect on the body

Adaptogens are nontoxic and, when consumed at normal therapeutic doses, are not associated with adverse side effects. This reflects an important tenet of natural medicine—*primum non nocere:* "First, do no harm."

These medicines are especially well-known for their ability to increase the body's resistance to physical, biological, chemical, environmental, and emotional stressors. They do this by way of a nonspecific action that affects a wide range of physiological, chemical, and biochemical factors. In this way, adaptogens work to keep the body healthy and balanced when faced with multiple stressors.

Adaptogens also work to increase or decrease various physiological functions to create balance and restore homeostasis in the body. In this way, adaptogens are able to correct functional imbalances in the body. For example, they can decrease activity in hyperfunctioning conditions or increase activity in hypofunctioning conditions. They act to adapt in ways that normalize function and resilience in the body.

These qualities help us handle stress more effectively at deep physiological, mental, and emotional levels. Adaptogens increase physical and mental endurance, reduce fatigue, combat chronic inflammation, enhance performance, improve cognitive function and mood, strengthen immune function, and promote vitality and longevity. They are especially helpful for treating conditions related to chronic stress, exhaustion, and depletion. They are considered anti-stress agents that energize and regenerate the body.

These medicinal plants and fungi also protect our cells from the damaging effects of stress, increase cellular energy production, regulate cellular metabolism, and enhance cellular function and survival. They have a normalizing effect and are able to restore both deficient and excess conditions back to their normal states. Taken together, all these qualities of adaptogens make them unique when compared to other pharmaceuticals, supplements, or even other botanicals.

An herb has to meet all of these criteria to be considered an adaptogen. The botanical adaptogens covered in this book all meet these criteria. These herbs will be discussed in more detail in chapter 2.

History

It is not known when adaptogens and other botanical medicines were first applied medicinally, but it seems their use predates written history. The oldest records of these herbs and fungi as medicines come from Chinese and Indian medicine and culture.

Cordyceps, licorice, Asian ginseng, eleuthero, and schisandra have been used for thousands of years in Chinese medicine. Written references to these botanical medicines have been found in some of the original Traditional Chinese Medicine textbooks. *Panax ginseng*, or Asian ginseng, was reputedly used by the Chinese mythological emperor Shennong and has been touted as an effective treatment for erectile function and sexual vitality.

The first written textbooks referencing medicinal plants in India date back to around 200 BCE. This ancient healing tradition is now known as Ayurveda, which means "the science of life." The best known of the traditional Ayurveda plants is holy basil, a sacred plant associated with the Hindu god Vishnu that is believed to nourish perfect health and longevity.

The modern uses of adaptogenic plants did not emerge until the 1940s. During World War II, the Soviet government instructed scientists to start looking for substances that could increase the physical performance of their soldiers, essentially in an effort to make "super soldiers." After World War II ended, this desire to find a substance that could improve performance and endurance, reduce fatigue, and improve mental function persisted through the onset of the Cold War. In an effort to create an edge against competitors, the search was on for a product that could increase the performance of their elite military personnel, political officers, athletes, and chess players.

In 1946, Russian physician Dr. Nikolai Lazarev started researching chemical substances that could fit these criteria. He began doing experiments with the chemical drug dibazol and discovered that when this drug was given to animals, it increased the animals' ability to resist stressors. Dr. Lazarev then officially coined the term *adaptogen* to describe these substances that could increase the general state of nonspecific resistance to stress.

One of his colleagues, Dr. Israel I. Brekhman, built on his work with synthetic adaptogens and began studying natural adaptogenic substances. Dr. Brekhman was involved in much of the early research into plant adaptogens, particularly *Eleutherococcus senticosus*, a plant native to Russia. Dr. Lazarev, Dr. Brekhman, and their team of scientists went on to study thousands more herbs, most notably rhodiola, schisandra, and rhaptonicum.

Adaptogens were used and studied for many years by the Russians to improve athletic performance in their Olympic athletes, train their astronauts, and improve the endurance and strength of their soldiers.

The Russians' work with adaptogens piqued the interest of the American Dr. Bruce W. Halstead. Dr. Halstead was the director of the World Life Research Institute in the United States and had been studying herbal medicine for many years. Dr. Halstead traveled to Russia, where he established a working relationship with the Soviet scientists. Upon his return to the United States, he introduced eleuthero to the American public under the name Siberian ginseng. He continued his research and published a book called *Eleutherococcus Senticosus (Siberian Ginseng): An Introduction to the Concept of Adaptogenic Medicine* in 1984. This book paved the way for its use and popularity in the United States.

Benefits

Use of adaptogens is increasing in popularity due to their incredible and widespread benefits for the mind and body. These benefits have been well documented and include promoting a healthy stress response, supporting energy and stamina, regulating metabolism, boosting immunity, supporting healing and regeneration, and promoting longevity and healthy aging (Panossian 2011).

Healthy Stress Response

Adaptogens are probably best known for their ability to promote a healthy stress response in the body. Our bodies help us cope with a range of physical, mental, emotional, and environmental stressors. Adaptogenic herbs can serve as essential allies as we navigate stresses large and small.

Adaptogens primarily work by regulating the HPA (hypothalamic-pituitary-adrenal) axis. They have the ability to "hack" into this axis to reregulate and normalize dysfunction. The health of the HPA axis is considered to be essential to a person's vitality, and disruption of the HPA axis is often the root cause of many chronic conditions.

When the body is stressed, the hypothalamus detects distress signals, then turns on a cascade of hormone signals (through the anterior pituitary) to stimulate the release of cortisol from the adrenal glands. In a normal healthy stress response, once the perceived threat has been controlled, cortisol then produces a negative feedback loop to the hypothalamus, signaling it to stop that cascade of hormone signals. However, in conditions of chronic stress, the hypothalamus is under continual attack and becomes desensitized to those negative feedback signals. Adaptogens help reregulate the stress response by restoring hypothalamic and pituitary sensitivity to the negative feedback of cortisol. This can turn off the constant pro-inflammatory effect of prolonged cortisol release and restore homeostasis in the function of the hypothalamus.

Hormone Balance

The HPA axis plays a significant role in the modulation of reproductive and sexual function through its effects on the HPG (hypothalamic-pituitary-gonadal) axis.

The HPG axis stimulates the production of estrogen, progesterone, and testosterone.

The HPA and HPG axes are closely connected. The action of one affects the function of the other. For example, estrogen and testosterone modulate the response of the HPA axis, and the HPA axis modulates the production of our sex hormones.

As mentioned previously, chronic stress continually activates the HPA axis. This leads to increased cortisol output and demand. In an attempt to keep up, the body steals pregnenolone, "the mother of hormones," away from the HPG axis and converts it into cortisol. Pregnenolone is a precursor to all sex hormones. This "pregnenolone steal" leads to the inhibition of estrogen, progesterone, and testosterone production, which can cause amenorrhea, symptoms associated with menopause, infertility, erectile dysfunction, loss of libido, and decreased sperm count.

Adaptogens modulate that stress response and therefore protect the HPG axis as well, restoring hormone balance in the body. Many adaptogens also have direct effects on the reproductive organs, acting as strengthening tonics and hormone regulators.

Energy and Stamina

Fatigue is one of the most common concerns that bring people to the doctor, and chronic stress is a common cause and contributing factor to physical, mental, and emotional fatigue. Adaptogens can help with all of those concerns.

Adaptogens help improve energy levels by boosting mitochondrial function. Mitochondria are the powerhouse organelles in our cells that produce energy in the form of adenosine triphosphate (ATP). Stress and intense physical activity increase the body's demands for ATP. Adaptogens help mitochondria keep up with those increased demands, resulting in increased energy, stamina, endurance, and muscle strength.

Adaptogens have also been shown to enhance cognitive function and improve mood by reducing mental and emotional fatigue. They have direct effects on the nervous system that combat stress-induced neuroinflammation, help improve sleep quality and duration, and regulate neurotransmitter levels.

Metabolism

Chronic stress affects our metabolism by disrupting thyroid function, blood sugar regulation, and the balance of metabolic biochemical processes.

Metabolism can be broadly broken down into two major mechanisms: anabolism and catabolism. Catabolism is a destructive mechanism that involves the breakdown of molecules. Anabolism does the opposite and involves the rebuilding of molecules. In a healthy state, these processes oppose each other in a harmonious balance. Chronic stress shifts this balance to favor catabolism, leading to repetitive destruction and wear and tear on the body. Adaptogens help restore the healthy balance.

The body's normal response to stress is to stimulate the release of glucose to provide the fuel it needs to effectively fight off a stressor. When glucose levels are high in the blood, insulin is released to lower blood sugar back into its normal range. Chronic stress can disrupt this normal response due to the continual release of glucocorticoids (stress hormones), which leads to blood sugar imbalances and insulin resistance. Adaptogens help regulate blood sugar levels by promoting a healthy glucocorticoid balance.

Excessive cortisol production can alter thyroid function by inhibiting the conversion of thyroid hormones into their active state. Thyroid hormones affect every cell in the body and regulate metabolism, cardiovascular function, digestion, body temperature, energy levels, and brain function. By normalizing the HPA axis, thyroid function can be optimized.

Immunity

Adaptogens work to restore and enhance function in the immune system in various ways. They regulate our body's stress response, modulate and strengthen immune function, decrease inflammation, and improve our body's resilience to stressors. Some adaptogens even have antiviral, antibacterial, and antitumor activity.

Adaptogens have immune-modulating functions. They are helpful at calming overactive immune states as well as stimulating immune function in deficient states.

Adaptogens increase production of immune cells, including B cells, T cells, and natural killer cells. These cells help the body fight off pathogens by killing foreign invaders, creating antibodies, and modulating the effect of other immune cells. Adaptogens also increase the production of cytokines, which are the immune system's chemical messenger cells. These cytokines (interleukin, TNF-alpha, and interferon) play a major role in modulating immune and inflammatory response to various pathogens in the body. Many chronic illnesses are associated with an unhealthy balance of cytokines. Adaptogens can correct these imbalances and restore harmony and resilience to the body.

Adaptogens are safe and effective treatments for autoimmune conditions, allergies, asthma, chronic infections, cancer, and many other imbalanced immune states.

Healing and Regeneration

Adaptogens promote healing and regeneration in the body through their ability to normalize and restore function. Adaptogens not only help the body mount the appropriate response to stressors but also help the body recover from those stressors.

Chronic stress alters HPA function and therefore creates imbalances in other systems in the body that are needed for recovery and regeneration. Stress is a common cause of sleep disturbances. During sleep, our bodies and our brains heal, regenerate, and recover. When our sleep is disrupted, our ability to fully heal is also disrupted. Adaptogens negate injurious stress responses and help reestablish healthy and restorative sleep.

Adaptogens also help our bodies heal and recover through their anti-inflammatory actions, enhancement of cellular detoxification, protection from stress-induced cellular destruction, and promotion of anabolic activities that work to restore and rebuild tissues. The ability to quickly recover from stressors was one of the advantages the Soviets were looking for to help their soldiers and athletes. They found this, and much more, in adaptogens.

Adaptogens possess the unique abilities to enhance HPA axis function and normalize function in the body. By helping bring the body back into homeostasis, adaptogens optimize the function of the immune, endocrine, and nervous systems, healing the body as a whole.

Longevity and Healthy Aging

There are many stress-related changes associated with aging, including inflammation, declining hormone levels, and an increase in catabolic processes and free radicals. Adaptogens can combat these adverse effects to enhance healthy aging and promote longevity.

As the body ages, its ability to maintain homeostasis under stress decreases. This results in a decline in our physical and mental health. Adaptogens can slow that decline through their ability to maintain homeostasis in the body.

Stress-induced inflammation plays a central role in the aging process. In a study published in *Frontiers in Immunology* in 2018, researchers found a profound increase in pro-inflammatory cytokine markers in many conditions associated with aging. Adaptogens are able to control this inflammatory response and maintain balance in immune function. Adaptogens have also been found to decrease inflammation on the cellular level by up-regulating molecular chaperones, protecting cells against stress-induced damage.

It has been proposed that another mechanism of aging is catabolic malfunction in the body. As discussed previously, catabolism is a destructive mechanism that can lead to increased cellular breakdown and loss of muscle mass. Adaptogens can restore anabolic activity to achieve a healthy metabolic balance.

Through these mechanisms, adaptogens promote healthy aging, vitality, and longevity.

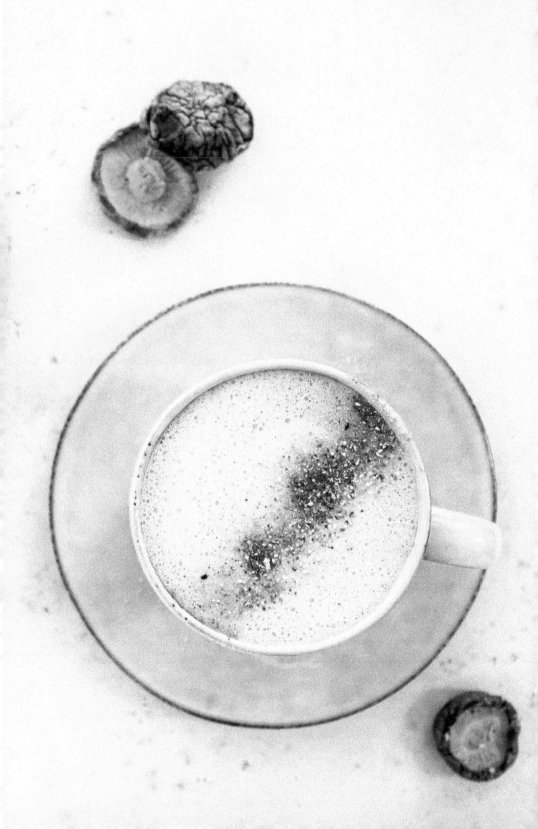

CHAPTER TWO

Nature's Stress Busters

Adaptogens are commonly referred to as nature's stress busters. These amazing botanicals help protect the body, mind, and spirit from the multitude of stressors that we face on a daily basis.

Stress-related concerns are the number one reason people seek professional help from a doctor, therapist, herbalist, or health consultant. This chapter explores some common stressors that affect us on a daily basis. If this chronic stress isn't mediated, it can lead to a myriad of neurological, endocrine, and detoxification imbalances in the body. Adaptogens can negate this stress response, allowing for optimal functioning of these systems. By returning the body to homeostasis and increasing its resilience, adaptogens help the body effectively fight off these stressors.

What Is Stress?

Modern-day humans are faced with an enormous amount of stress on a daily basis. When most people think about stress, they picture a state of emotional and physical fatigue. Unfortunately though, anything that our bodies perceive as a threat can be a stressor. This can include biological, physical, chemical, nutritional, psychological, and spiritual stress. These stressors disrupt the body's internal balance through their effects on the hypothalamus, the key mediator of the body.

Work Stress

We live in a society where achievement, success, and productivity are top priorities.

Increased work demands, excessive responsibilities, constant deadlines, worry about professional performance, and financial struggles are common stresses that many people face on a daily basis. These stresses can quickly lead to burnout and adversely affect our mood, sleep, and physical health.

Technology and Stress

Although technological advances have their benefits, they also have their downfalls. Easy access to the news, social media, and email allows our brains to be constantly engaged. This continuous stimulation unconsciously sends the brain into stress mode, making it hard to unwind and de-stress from the day. The lights that are emitted from these electronics also inhibit our melatonin production, altering our normal sleep-wake cycle and affecting our quality of sleep.

Insufficient sleep is one of the biggest obstacles to restoring a person's health and well-being. I often work with patients on improving their sleep hygiene, limiting use of electronics, and spending more time in nature. These lifestyle modifications, along with the use of adaptogenic herbs, help restore the body's normal circadian rhythm and resilience.

Psychological and Spiritual Stress

Fear, anger, sadness, grief, disappointment, worry, and the feeling of being overwhelmed can all elicit our stress response. Although these are all normal human emotions, they still take their toll on the body. When these emotions are experienced on a regular basis, they add significantly to the chronic stress load of the mind and body.

Misalignments in our values and beliefs can cause psychospiritual stress and disrupt our sense of self and authenticity. Feeling disconnected, questioning faith, losing a sense of purpose, or struggling with self-love all put unwanted stress on the spiritual psyche. Empirical studies have shown a positive correlation between a person's spirituality and health. Holistic health care recognizes the spiritual self as an integral part of the whole person and can help fix these misalignments in a person's life. Holy basil is a wonderful plant for helping with this type of stress, as this adaptogen is especially well-known for its spiritual healing abilities.

Food and Diet

In naturopathic medicine, a healthy diet is considered to be an essential aspect of a person's health. The body requires food to survive, and the types of food we put in our bodies affect how they function. Many foods that are common in the standard American diet are pro-inflammatory and devoid of adequate nutrition, resulting in increased stress and toxic load on the body.

Fast foods, processed foods, trans fats, refined carbohydrates, food additives and dyes, sugar, alcohol, allergenic foods, and pesticide-loaded produce all wreak havoc on our digestive tracts and trigger the release of those inflammatory cytokines we previously talked about (see page 11). Regular consumption of these pro-inflammatory foods results in a constant state of stress on the body, negatively affecting our digestion and detoxification pathways.

Environmental Toxins

The average person is exposed to a plethora of toxins on a daily basis. Chemicals, pesticides, heavy metals, pharmaceuticals, plastics, mold, air pollution . . . unfortunately, the list is endless. Toxins are also commonly found in cleaning products, personal care products, and even in the food and water we eat and drink. These environmental toxins create stress and inflammation in the body and impair our detoxification pathways. As a result, these toxins build up in the body and contribute to many chronic health conditions. Many of these toxins are also endocrine, immune, and neurological disrupters, directly affecting these body systems.

Physical Stress

Physical stressors can include acute injuries or trauma, pain, strenuous physical activity, and underlying health conditions. The body's normal response to acute injury or pain is an inflammatory and immune response to fight off the injury and stimulate the healing process. When the body is under repetitive or chronic pain or trauma, this inflammatory response goes unchecked, adding to systemic inflammation.

Biological Stress

Biological stressors include any exposure to foreign bacteria, viruses, fungi, or parasites. These stressors elicit an immunological and stress response to fight off the pathogenic invaders. When the body is stressed, its immune function is unbalanced. This altered immune function can lead to auto-immune or lowered immune states.

Current Events and Stress

The year 2020 posed significant stressors for many people. At the time that this book is being written, people worldwide are facing an extremely contagious viral infection known as COVID-19. Not only has this virus presented significant health challenges for many people—it has also spiked anxieties regarding social and financial struggles. Social distancing has been mandated in many countries, forcing people to isolate from friends and family. Parents are juggling work, childcare, and the uncertainty of remote learning. People are losing their jobs, companies are being forced to shut down, and the economy as a whole is struggling. Worst of all, many people have become seriously ill and have tragically lost their lives. The grief and emotional toll that this virus has inflicted on us will likely remain long after this pandemic has been contained. Now more than ever, people need additional support for their health and healing.

The Neuroendocrine System

The nervous and endocrine systems are intricately connected and commonly referred to together as the neuroendocrine system. The neuroendocrine system is composed of many auto-regulatory systems consisting of multiple hormonal feedback loops that provide input to the brain. The HPA axis is central to hormonal regulation and the function of the neuroendocrine system.

The hypothalamus is the key regulator of the neuroendocrine system. It controls the release of chemical messengers to the anterior pituitary, which then regulates the release of our thyroid hormones, steroid hormones, growth hormones, and sex hormones. When the body is in homeostasis, these hormones remain in a balanced, harmonious state. Stress, however, can be a major disrupter of endocrine function and homeostatic balance. When the hypothalamus detects something it perceives as a threat, it releases hormones to activate a stress response.

There are three phases of the stress response: the alarm phase, the resistance phase, and the exhaustion phase. Most of what we have discussed so far has been related to the resistance and exhaustion phases. These are where HPA stress and depletion occur and where most individuals remain after exposure to chronic stress. Adaptogens are most helpful for recovering from these stages.

The first part of the initial stress response is referred to as the alarm phase. This response is dominated by the autonomic nervous system, which is comprised of the sympathetic and parasympathetic nervous systems. Our sympathetic nervous system activates our first act of defense against a stressor, commonly known as our "fight or flight" response.

When the hypothalamus detects a stressor, it signals the spinal cord to activate the autonomic stress response and the anterior pituitary to activate the secretion of adrenocorticotropic hormone (ACTH) and subsequent cortisol release (HPA axis response). The sympathetic nervous system then stimulates our adrenal gland to release epinephrine and norepinephrine to set off the alarm. The ensuing sympathetic state increases heart rate and blood pressure, accelerates respiration rate, shunts blood flow from our core into our extremities, and raises blood sugar. These reactions are meant to fuel our bodies with the necessary energy needed to "run from the bear" and away from danger. In this alarm phase, interleukin-6 and C-reactive protein (inflammatory cytokines) are also quickly released to cause a pro-inflammatory response.

The resistance phase is when the body attempts to resist these stressors and return to homeostasis. In this stage, the parasympathetic nervous system works to counteract the sympathetic nervous system and pull our bodies out of the chronic inflammatory stress response. When the HPA axis is optimally functioning, cortisol release will be turned off when the stressor has been removed, and the body will return to homeostasis.

However, under conditions of persistent or repeated stress, the body remains in a chronically elevated cortisol state. This causes widespread inflammation and over time desensitizes the body and brain to the effects of cortisol. This not only leads to HPA axis dysfunction but also adversely affects hormone regulation and endocrine function.

These prolonged states of elevated cortisol levels inhibit the endocrine pathways that regulate our thyroid, melatonin, pancreatic, and sex hormone production. This can lead to thyroid disorders, male and female hormonal imbalances, sexual dysfunction, infertility, sleep disorders, insulin resistance, and other metabolic issues.

If the body persists in this resistance stage for too long, it can lead to the exhaustion stage. The exhaustion stage is a result of prolonged or chronic stress. In this stage, our bodies lose the ability to effectively resist stress, and we are more susceptible to disease. This is commonly known as "burnout."

Adaptogens can pull us out of the resistance and exhaustion phases by modulating the cortisol response, reestablishing normal HPA function, and restoring endocrine balance. A healthy, functioning HPA axis then promotes optimal functioning of the neuroendocrine system as a whole.

Detoxification Pathways

We live in a toxic world, and we all have some level of environmental toxic exposure. By enhancing your body's detoxification pathways and thus cleansing the body, you can reduce your toxic body burden and relieve any symptoms of toxicity you may be experiencing. Detoxification can also improve your long-term health and reduce your risk of chronic disease.

The liver is our primary detoxification organ. There are two main detoxification pathways. Phase 1 of liver detoxification is the first line of defense against toxins. A group of enzymes known as the cytochrome P450 pathway catalyze various chemical reactions (oxidation, reduction, and hydrolysis) that convert toxic substances into less-harmful molecules. During this process, free radicals are produced. If toxic exposure is high and a large number of free radicals are produced, liver cells can become damaged.

Phase 2 of liver detoxification is known as the conjugation phase. The main function of this phase is to further convert toxic substances into water-soluble molecules that can be easily eliminated from the body.

Stress can affect liver detoxification in many ways. Many environmental stressors, such as pesticides, can cause overactivation of the cytochrome P450 pathways. If the free radicals produced in Phase 1 are not quickly passed through to the Phase 2 pathway, cellular damage and increased toxic by-products may occur. This increased inflammation and toxicity just adds more fuel to the fire by causing more stress in the body.

Psychophysiological stress has also been shown to affect liver detoxification by up-regulating some cytochrome enzymes and down-regulating others. As most pharmaceuticals are metabolized through the cytochrome P450 pathway, stress can affect the pharmacokinetics of many drugs. Altering this drug metabolism can result in either reduced effectiveness or increased side effects and toxicity.

Adaptogens can help with liver detoxification by decreasing the effects of stressors on liver metabolism. Many adaptogens are also hepatoprotectants, which serve to protect the liver against damage. Hepatoprotective herbs can enhance liver function, help regenerate liver cells, and increase levels of glutathione, a powerhouse antioxidant and major detoxifying agent in the body. Schisandra is an excellent hepatoprotective adaptogen and should be considered the go-to botanical for individuals with liver sluggishness due to stress.

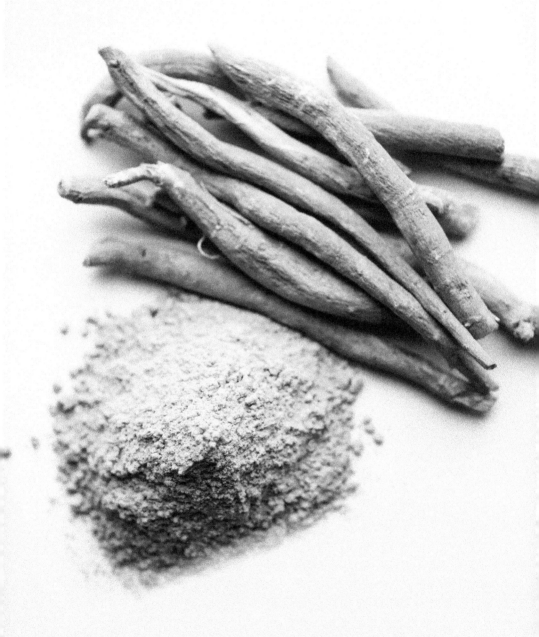

CHAPTER THREE

How to Use Adaptogens

There are many things to consider when it comes to using adaptogen herbs. This chapter explores the myriad considerations involved in safely and effectively dosing them for children and adults, and the various preparations of these botanicals.

Herbal purity, potency, and quality are essential aspects of botanical medicines. Extensive testing is required when manufacturing herbal products to ensure this purity and quality. We will discuss what questions to ask and what to look for when sourcing your herbs to ensure this safety.

Once you have determined how to safely and effectively use your herbs, it can be helpful to track your health progress in a journal in order to maintain accountability and achieve your health goals.

Sourcing Adaptogens

Love, intent, knowledge, and respect should go into harvesting and manufacturing plant medicine. Sustainable herbal practices help protect plants and fungi from becoming overharvested and endangered. They also help maintain biodiversity and the health of the soil and earth. These practices include cover crop rotation, herbal crop rotation, soil building, and biodiversity management. A cover crop is a crop that you grow to enrich the soil, as these crops add organic matter and nutrients. Crop rotation involves moving plants to different locations each year to prevent them from depleting nutrients in the soil. These are all important practices for growing plants, as healthy plants need healthy soil to thrive. A "green herbalist" recognizes the importance of these practices and provides a reliable source for obtaining herbs.

It's important to know where your herbs are coming from and how they were grown. You want to look for products that have been organically grown or wild harvested. Validate herb purity and potency as well. Herbs should be tested for impurities and have gone through a variety of other testing methods to ensure product quality and authenticity. If you are not sure about your herbs, I encourage you to ask the herbal companies or local growers who produce them these questions. If they are following these quality-assurance steps, they will be happy and proud to answer your questions. If they refuse or don't know how to answer, that is a red flag. You can also ask manufacturers to show you the results of their contaminant and potency testing for further assurance.

When you are buying herbs in the store, I encourage you to shop at local health food stores and co-ops, as they tend to carry reliable herbal products. When shopping online, try to seek out professional herbal companies that specialize in botanical supplements instead of shopping on more general e-commerce sites. I am always wary of buying supplements and herbs from third-party vendors, as you cannot verify the original source or quality of a product, even if it may be labeled with a popular brand name. Please refer to the Resources section (see page 146) of this book for recommendations on where to find quality herbal products online.

Ensuring Safety and Efficacy

To ensure safety and efficacy when using botanical medicine, it is important to consider the appropriate dosing recommendations for each plant, how to store your herbs, and what individualizing factors to examine when choosing your herbs.

More is not necessarily better when it comes to botanicals. Although adaptogens have a relatively high safety profile, there are other herbal medicines that are considered low-dose and cannot be taken in dosages higher than what is recommended. Special care should be taken when giving herbs to children, as the dosing recommendations for children are much lower than they are for adults.

Storing your herbs properly is just as important as obtaining high-quality herbal products. Proper storage methods will help ensure the maximum potency and continued purity of your herbs.

Dosing Guidelines

Although adaptogen herbs are typically very safe, it is recommended to follow the specific dosing guidelines for each herb. These dosing guidelines ensure safety and allow for the therapeutic benefits to be achieved. However, it is also important to consider other factors such as the age, weight, and constitutional strength of an individual. For example, the dosage for children of any particular herb will be much lower than the dosage for adults. Elderly individuals may also need a lower dose due to impaired digestive and detoxification functions. The use of pharmaceutical medications may also alter dosages due to the effect of such medications on liver detoxification pathways. Working with a knowledgeable physician or herbalist will ensure the most appropriate dosing recommendations in these circumstances.

People who tend to be very sensitive to medications and other supplements should also start with low and slow dosing of herbs. It is recommended these individuals try single herbs first to better assess tolerance.

Herbs are best taken on an empty stomach and in divided doses throughout the day. It is recommended to consume stimulating adaptogens in the morning and relaxing adaptogens later in the day.

Herbs for Children

Herbs make excellent treatment options for kids. However, they only work if you can get a child to take them. I see a lot of children in my clinical practice, and I have learned a few good tricks for getting herbs into kids.

Many herbs can be formulated into a glycerin or syrup. This adds sweetness to the flavor that most children enjoy. If that's not enough, adding another sweet-tasting herb such as elderberry can help. Powdered herbs can also be used and are easily hidden in applesauce, juice, smoothies, or pureed foods.

It's important to note that many of the pediatric herbal syrup formulas found over the counter contain honey. Honey cannot be given to children under the age of one due to the risk of botulism, which causes weakness and loss of muscle tone and can be fatal. Because of this concern, it is very important to check your labels, as formulas containing honey must be avoided for children under the age of one. For children over the age of one, though, they make yummy medicine options.

Teas also make excellent botanical options for children, as they are gentle and can be easily diluted to tolerance and sweetened up with honey or fruit juice. Another fun way to use teas is to freeze them into popsicles, which provides a refreshing summer treat.

Herbal baths, compresses, and topical salves and ointments are also great ways for getting herbs into children*, especially for those picky kids who refuse to take most medicines.

Pediatric doses can be determined by following a few different formulas:

Clark's Rule: child's weight in pounds/150 pounds × the adult dose = child's dose

Young's Rule: child's age/(child's age + 12) × the adult dose = child's dose

Only for children age 2 and over

It is most reliable and accurate to calculate the correct dosage for a child based on their individual weight, which is why Clark's Rule is the preferred method of dosing. For children under the age of one, it is best to consult a physician or herbalist trained in using herbs with children.

Storage Considerations

Just like all plants, adaptogenic herbs need the right environment to thrive. However, the needs of dried botanicals are very different from the needs of wild plants. Although we naturally think of sunlight, open air, and water as essential for gardening, dried herbs have the exact opposite requirements. Heat, light, moisture, and air can deteriorate dried herbs. To best protect dried botanicals from those elements, it is recommended to store them in cool, dry, dark, and airtight containers. Dark amber jars with tight-fitting lids work well for this. When buying herbs at the store, it is also important to note how they are packaged. If dried herbs are stored in clear, light-exposed containers, the quality will not be the same. If you are packaging your own herbs, it is best to encapsulate the freshly made powders as soon as possible to limit the damage from oxygenation and light exposure.

Herbs in tincture form have relatively long and stable shelf lives and do not need to be stored as carefully as dried herbs.

It's important to take note of the manufactured and expiration dates if you are buying herbs over the counter. Whereas most herbal preparations just lose potency over time, certain preparations such as glycerin formulas should not be used at all past their expiration dates as they may become a hospitable environment for microbes and mold.

Choosing an Application

There are many wonderful ways to enjoy adaptogenic plants and fungi. They can be used in tincture, tea, powder, capsule, topical, or edible form. Each of these application methods has their own advantages and disadvantages. We will discuss each one to help you determine which may be best for you and your needs.

Tinctures

Tinctures, also known as liquid extracts, are comprised of alcohol and water preparations of an herb. Tinctures provide several advantages over other preparations. Alcohol is a much better solvent than water and allows nearly all the herbal constituents to be extracted. Thus, tinctures are generally considered to provide the strongest and most concentrated dose of a plant. Herbs in tincture form are highly bioavailable, providing increased assimilation.

Alcohol is also a preservative, increasing the shelf life and stability of the herbal medicine. The typical shelf life of liquid extract tinctures is four to six years. The amount of alcohol in this liquid extract form is minimal, but if alcohol is not suitable for an individual, it can be evaporated by adding the herbal drops to a cup of boiling water.

Tinctures can also be made without alcohol. The substitutes for alcohol include vegetable glycerin and vinegar. Vegetable glycerin is commonly used to prepare children's herbs. Glycerin preparations have the advantage of improving taste by adding sweetness to the herbal concoction. One disadvantage of glycerin preparations is that their shelf life is relatively short at 12 to 24 months.

When measuring tinctures, keep in mind that 1 milliliter is equal to 1 dropperful.

Capsules and Powders

Herbs can also be ground into a powder, but this gives them a much shorter shelf life, as they are more susceptible to the effects of light, heat, and oxygen in this form. Because of this, powdered herbs should be used immediately so that they are as fresh as possible. Powdered herbs are often used for capsules, teas, and suppository application. They can make a great option for children, as they can be easily hidden in food.

Capsules provide a convenient way to consume herbal medicines while reducing the herbal taste that some people do not like. They often increase compliance with prescriptions due to the fact that they are easier to take and travel with. Herbs can be encapsulated from either dried or liquid extract preparations. Powdered encapsulations of dried herbs are the most common. The disadvantages of encapsulated dried herbs are that they generally have less activity and digestibility than liquid forms.

In 2001, Gaia Herbs, one of the leading growers and producers of certified organic herbs and herbal products, introduced liquid phyto-capsules. This patented delivery of liquid extracts combines the advantages of encapsulated and tincture botanical applications.

Teas

Teas are an enjoyable way to consume adaptogens. Teas are best used in fresh preparations and can be easily made by steeping dried herbs in boiling water. Taking herbs in this way also allows you to easily control the strength of each herbal dose, giving you a more empowered role in the process.

Teas make an effective treatment option for individuals who may need a gentler or reduced dose of medicine. They are quicker to digest and thus easier on the weakened digestive states that may be found in elderly or young individuals.

Teas can be especially useful as part of your stress-reduction regimen, since just the act of sitting and drinking a cup of tea can be healing. This ritual forces us to take the time to slow down in a very fast-paced world. Drinking teas as part of your nighttime regimen can be helpful for promoting healthy sleep hygiene and reminding your brain that it is preparing for sleep.

A downside to teas is that they are best when immediately consumed, which requires more time, effort, and accountability from the individual. The shelf life of dried herbs is not as long as that of tinctures with many dried herbs only lasting for about a year. Dried herbs can also take up more space in the kitchen, which may be a disadvantage for people with limited kitchen space.

Edibles and Topicals

The oldest traditional use of botanicals involved eating and cooking with the plants. Asian ginseng roots were chewed to enhance male sexual function and vitality. Other adaptogens were cooked into foods as a delicacy.

Adaptogens and other botanicals are still commonly used in these ways. Medicinal mushrooms are one of the more popular edible versions of plant medicine. Adaptogenic fungi, such as cordyceps, can be easily cooked with your favorite vegetables to provide a delicious and enjoyable way to get your daily adaptogen dose. Root adaptogens such as ashwagandha and ginseng can be cooked into stews or broths.

Herbs have also commonly been used in topical forms throughout herbal history and can be applied through poultices, healing salves, ointments, baths, compresses, and essential oils. Topical applications are most commonly used to heal wounds and infections and to soothe skin irritation and inflammation. Adaptogens typically are not used in topical applications, as internal use of these herbs is most effective. However, licorice root extract is an exception to that rule due to its potent antiviral and anti-inflammatory effects and is commonly found in many topical herbal formulas.

Spirit Dosing and Homeopathic Preparations

Spirit dosing is a way to seek out the emotional and spiritual energetics of plant medicine. It involves taking very small doses of herbs to extract more of their energetic qualities. This dosing typically consists of only a few drops (one to five) of plant extracts and is often suggested for individuals who are struggling with psychological and spiritual stressors.

Spirit dosing can be helpful in treating grief, trauma, apathy, loss of purpose in one's life, or feelings of disconnectedness. It may also be used in very sensitive individuals who do not tolerate normal therapeutic doses of medications, supplements, or herbal medicines.

Another way to seek out the spiritual energetics of herbs is through herbal bathing. Spiritual herbal baths are often used to refresh and purify the body. The power and healing properties of water and medicinal plants can provide deep cleansing and spiritual renewal at an energetic level.

Meditation, prayer, and other spiritual practices can also increase the energetic and spiritual benefits provided from these healing herbs.

Tracking Results

You will get the most benefit out of adaptogenic herbs by working with an herbalist. A professional can help tailor an individual treatment plan and health program for you. Once this treatment plan is created, it is helpful to create a health journal to record your progress.

I often recommend health journals to my patients, as they are excellent educational tools that help you learn more about your health and your body. These journals can be especially helpful when assessing diet and lifestyle patterns and tracking symptoms. Our dietary and lifestyle habits often directly contribute to our digestive issues, brain fog, fatigue, and many other imbalances. Tracking these symptoms in a health journal can increase awareness of our bodies and what may be affecting them. This can serve as a valuable investigative tool for determining the root causes of your symptoms. Once you have identified any potential obstacles to your health, you will be able to tackle them more effectively.

When beginning any new treatment program, it is helpful to note when you start a new herb or supplement, as well as what application and dose you use. Tracking the changes you notice physically and psychologically on a new herbal regimen will help you determine which herbs, doses, and applictions are most beneficial to you.

If you're new to plant medicine, it is recommended to start low and slow with one botanical at a time. This allows you to understand which herbs are most beneficial to you and how individual herbs affect you. Experimenting with different botanicals and herbal preparation methods also adds fun and enjoyment to your healing regimen. You may find a certain herbal preparation calls to your spirit more, or that certain tastes do not fit your palate as well.

The information in this book can help you determine when these various botanical preparations and individual herbs may be more useful in different circumstances in your life. This is part of the beauty of using herbal medicine and something I believe you will enjoy. As you become more familiar with these powerhouse plants, you will learn to appreciate how amazing they really are. This may lead you to experiment with other complementary botanicals, such as nervines, which are herbs that are nourishing to the nervous system, and restorative tonics. Some examples of these botanicals will be discussed in chapter 5. (Many adaptogens also act as nervines, and all adaptogens function as restorative tonics to the body.)

Creating your own health journal also empowers you to take more responsibility in your health care. I have learned that the more active people are in making their own decisions, the more motivated they are to make lasting changes to improve their health. I regularly help my patients find these motivations and maintain accountability. Educating people on how things like stress affect their bodies helps them understand why these stress-reducing interventions are so essential.

As with any treatment regimen, it is important to remember to practice forgiveness, as we are often our worst critics. An occasional indulgence in comfort food or a missed workout does not equate to failure in your treatment program and health goals. These are all normal tendencies that just mean you are human. It's also important to not just rely on the power of adaptogens to restore health and resilience in the body. If you're constantly subjecting your body to emotional, physical, and nutritional stresses, these herbs will only act as a bandage on a deeper, underlying problem. You will receive the most benefit from these herbs when they are used alongside a healthy diet, exercise, and stress-reduction practices.

The best part of using a health journal is that by documenting your progress you can look back to where you were and how far you have come. The changes you see in your life may include increased productivity at work, more energy, better sleep, happier mood, and reduced feelings of stress. Restoring your health and vitality is a rewarding experience. Having evidence that reminds you of your accomplishments will help you continue to live a life of resilience.

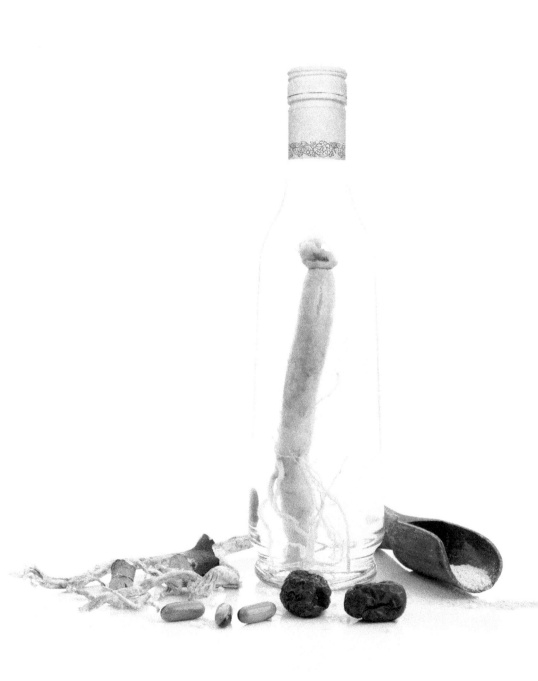

PART TWO

Discover and Heal

This section of the book will explore several adaptogenic plants and fungi, as well as other botanical allies that complement their actions.

The adaptogenic plants and fungi discussed here were chosen because they are nontoxic, produce a nonspecific response to stress, and have a normalizing and balancing effect on the body. They have been well researched and are commonly used in modern practice.

We will explore several health concerns that can be treated with adaptogen and complementary herbs. We will also discuss how to best enhance your herbal treatment regimen with healthy lifestyle practices that reduce stress, enhance stamina, and ease dis-ease.

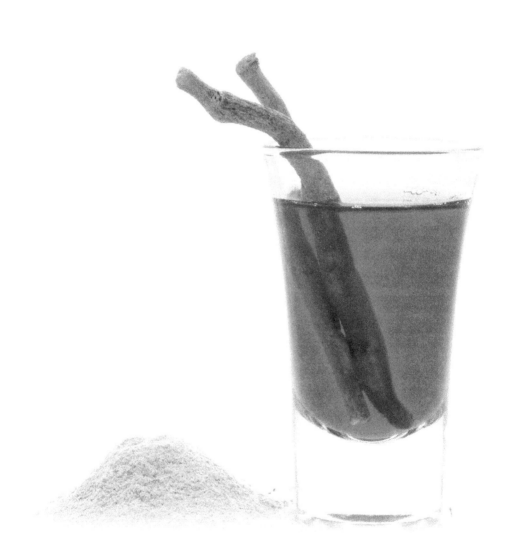

CHAPTER FOUR

Classic Adaptogens

The adaptogens in this chapter are considered our all-stars because of their stress-busting, immune-modulating, energy-enhancing, and mood-boosting effects. These adaptogens normalize HPA axis function and support optimal neuroendocrine health. They can be used to achieve wellness, vitality, and longevity.

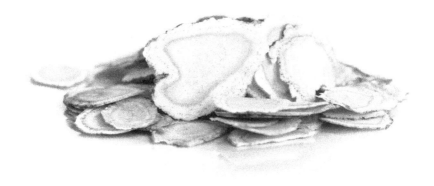

American Ginseng

LATIN NAME: *Panax quinquefolius*

American ginseng is one of two adaptogenic plants native to North America. (Rhodiola [see page 87] is the other.) It is native to the northeastern parts of the United States and Canada. Due to overharvesting, wild American ginseng is unfortunately endangered in many areas.

American ginseng was used for its medicinal properties long before the United States was founded. Indigenous Americans commonly consumed it to treat digestive troubles, pain, respiratory issues, and fatigue and to improve brain function and sexual vitality. It was believed to be a cure-all.

This adaptogen is very similar in its actions to that of its relative Asian ginseng (see page 47). However, American ginseng is more moistening, less warm and stimulating, and more active on the digestive tract. It is considered a mild digestive tonic and stimulant. American ginseng is especially helpful to individuals with mental and nervous exhaustion, loss of appetite, and digestive issues.

American Ginseng at a Glance

HELPFUL PARTS: root

ADDITIONAL NAMES: sang, seng, xi yang shen

COMMON PREPARATIONS: capsules, decoction (mashing up the plant material and boiling it to extract the beneficial oils and chemical compounds for use in tinctures, teas, and cooking), dried root/crude plant, tincture

ENERGETICS AND TASTE: bitter, moist, sweet, warm. Decreases Vatta and increases Pitta and Kapha. Taken in small doses, it is tridoshic (balancing to the three Ayurvedic states).

MEDICINAL PROPERTIES: adaptogenic, cardioprotective, circulation enhancer, digestive tonic, hepatoprotective, hypoglycemic/insulin sensitizing, hypolipidemic, immune-modulating, stimulant, tonic, tumor inhibitor

IDEAL FOR ADDRESSING: adrenal fatigue, athletic performance, brain fog/poor memory, cancer prevention and treatment, cardiovascular health, erectile dysfunction, immunity, male infertility, peak performance, weakness/debility

Benefits

ENERGY AND VITALITY: American ginseng is extremely helpful for treating HPA axis dysregulation and adrenal fatigue. It is indicated for individuals with mental, emotional, and physical exhaustion; chronic stress, disrupted sleep; and elevated cortisol levels. As an adaptogen, American ginseng increases the resistance to physical, chemical, and biological stressors and improves HPA axis function.

It is well-known for its ability to reduce fatigue, improve mental and physical performance, and enhance vitality.

DIGESTIVE FUNCTION: American ginseng was traditionally well-known for its tonifying and strengthening actions on the digestive tract. It is a stimulating digestive bitter that enhances digestion and nutrient absorption. It is useful for treating digestive concerns related to low stomach acid production, and the root itself can be chewed on to stimulate digestive juices.

ENDOCRINE AND IMMUNE AMPHOTERIC (BALANCER): American ginseng can modulate and regulate normal immune function. It is helpful for treating allergies, allergic asthma, autoimmune conditions, and immune deficiency. Its moistening effects make it especially useful for treating dry immune conditions such as Sjogren's syndrome.

BLOOD SUGAR REGULATION: American ginseng's effects on the HPA axis help control blood sugar, insulin resistance, and type 2 diabetes.

MALE SEXUAL FUNCTION: Like its relative, Asian ginseng (see page 47), American ginseng is well-known for its ability to enhance male sexual function and balance reproductive hormones. It is commonly used in the treatment of erectile dysfunction.

How to Use American Ginseng

American ginseng is popularly used in tincture, capsule, and tea form. The root can be cooked and added to medicinal soups or broths.

Recommended Amounts

CAPSULES (POWDERED HERB): 400 to 500 milligrams, 2 or 3 times per day

CRUDE PLANT: 5 to 10 grams per day

DECOCTION: 1 teaspoon to 1 tablespoon of dried root (cut and sifted) per 1 to 1½ cups of water. Simmer for 30 minutes, then steep for an additional half hour. Drink ½ cup, 2 or 3 times a day.

TINCTURE (1:2): 1 to 3 milliliters, 2 to 3 times per day

TINCTURE (1:5): 2 to 5 milliliters, 2 to 3 times per day

Cautions and Considerations

This adaptogen is relatively safe when properly dosed. It may increase the effects of blood-thinning medication due to its blood-thinning actions.

Recipes

Ginseng has been used in Chinese medicinal cooking for many centuries. The root can be eaten raw or cooked into stews and broths.

Chicken Soup with a Zing

SERVES 8 | Prep time: 10 minutes | Cook time: 2 to 3 hours

This recipe can be used to boost your immune system, strengthen your adrenal glands, support digestive and reproductive health, and nourish your soul.

1 (3-pound) whole chicken
2 American ginseng roots
4 organic carrots
4 organic celery stalks
1 large organic onion
2 tablespoons chopped
  fresh parsley

1 tablespoon chopped
  fresh rosemary
1 tablespoon chopped
  fresh thyme
1 to 2 tablespoons peeled grated
  fresh ginger (optional)

1. In a large soup pot, combine the chicken and ginseng and cover with water by about an inch. Simmer, uncovered, for about an hour, then add the carrots, celery, and onion. Continue to cook for another 1 to 2 hours, until the chicken meat falls off the bones and the vegetables are tender. The longer you simmer, the richer the flavor. Remove from heat and take the chicken, vegetables, and ginseng out of the pot.
2. Pick the chicken off the bones and shred. Chop the carrots, celery, and onion into bite-size pieces. Discard the ginseng. Return the chicken and vegetables back to the broth.
3. Add the parsley, rosemary, thyme, and ginger (if using). Stir together for 3 to 5 minutes, then serve warm. Enjoy 1 to 2 servings per day. Store leftovers in an airtight container in the refrigerator for up to 5 days.

Adrenal Restoration Tincture

MAKES 120 MILLILITERS (4 OUNCES)
Prep time: 2 minutes

The herbs in this formula boost energy, enhance stamina, strengthen the immune system, and restore function to the adrenal glands. You should notice immediate improvements in your energy after using this tincture, but for more lasting results this formula should be taken for at least 2 months.

40 milliliters American ginseng (1:2)
30 milliliters eleuthero (1:2)

25 milliliters *Glycyrrhiza glabra* (1:2)
25 milliliters cordyceps (1:4)

1. Using a funnel, measure the American ginseng, eleuthero, *Glycyrrhiza glabra*, and cordyceps tinctures in a graduated cylinder, then transfer to a 4-ounce glass bottle.
2. Take a dose of 3 to 4 milliliters 2 times per day, mid-morning and early afternoon between meals.

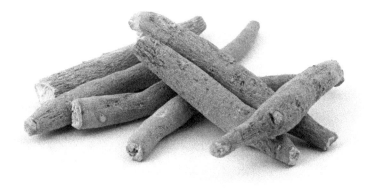

Ashwagandha

LATIN NAME: *Withania somnifera*

Ashwagandha can be found wild in the southern and central dry regions of Asia and Africa. It is an erect shrub that grows up to 1 meter tall with leaves that grow up to 10 centimeters in length. This plant produces yellow-green flowers that develop into berries.

The name *ashwagandha* means "the smell of a horse" in Sanskrit. This describes the plant well, as ashwagandha is known to increase vitality, strength, and stamina. It is especially helpful for people who are exhausted and agitated from chronic stress. Ashwagandha is both reinvigorating and restorative to the body and mind. It has a calming effect on the nervous system and also supports thyroid function and male health.

In Ayurvedic medicine, ashwagandha is classified as a rasayana, which is similar to an adaptogen. Rasayanas are plants that promote physical and mental health, augment the body's resistance to disease, restore and revitalize the body, and promote longevity.

Ashwagandha at a Glance

HELPFUL PARTS: root

ADDITIONAL NAMES: Indian ginseng, winter cherry

COMMON PREPARATIONS: capsules, decoction, tincture

ENERGETICS AND TASTE: astringent, bitter, heating, "smell of a horse," sweet

MEDICINAL PROPERTIES: adaptogenic, anti-anxiolytic, anti-inflammatory, antitumor, antioxidant, boosts fertility, enhances sexual function, immune-modulating, memory enhancing, nervine, supports thyroid function

IDEAL FOR ADDRESSING: signs of aging, anxiety, brain fog, chronic stress, infertility, insomnia, low energy and vitality, low immune function, low libido, low thyroid function, male sexual function

Benefits

THYROID FUNCTION: Ashwagandha is one of the few herbs that acts directly on the thyroid gland. It is stimulating to thyroid function and can be helpful in mild cases of hypothyroidism. It is safe to use in conjunction with thyroid medication and works wonderfully as a complementary herb. Ashwagandha is especially useful for support-ing the treatment of Hashimoto's disease, an autoimmune thyroid condition. This is due to its adaptogenic, immune-modulating, and anti-inflammatory effects.

Many modern-day stresses, such as emotional stress and exposure to environmental toxins, affect thyroid function. As an adaptogen, ashwagandha helps support thyroid function by reducing the effects of these stressors on the thyroid gland. Ashwagandha also helps reduce common symptoms of hypothyroidism, such as brain fog and fatigue.

MALE SEXUAL FUNCTION: In Ayurvedic medicine, one of the more traditional uses of ashwagandha has been as a male tonic and sexual enhancer. Ashwagandha supports male fertility by increasing sperm count and motility and reproductive hormones like testosterone. Ashwagandha repairs oxidative stress, which is a major factor in male and female infertility. Studies have shown that ashwagandha actually increases antioxidant levels in sperm. It is used in Ayurvedic medicine to treat erectile dysfunction, but clinical studies have not validated the efficacy of this usage. Ashwagandha supports a healthy sex drive in men and is believed to give men the "strength of a stallion."

BRAIN AND COGNITIVE HEALTH: Ashwagandha is a calming adaptogen and nervine. It is nourishing to the nervous system and especially helpful in "wired and tired" conditions like anxiety, insomnia, and nervous exhaustion. It also helps clear foggy thinking and enhances memory and brain function.

Ashwagandha binds to GABA receptors in the brain, promoting a calming GABAergic effect that lessens anxiety and can even help reduce cravings from morphine drug withdrawal.

Somnifera, from the plant's Latin name, means "sleep making." Ashwagandha helps restore normal sleep patterns in those who experience insomnia as a result of chronic stress.

IMMUNE FUNCTION: Ashwagandha can increase red and white blood cell counts in people who are anemic, exhausted, or immune-depleted. It can be used as a safe, complementary treatment to chemotherapy. Ashwagandha also has antitumor activity and has been shown to help decrease tumor number and size.

Ashwagandha is strengthening and balancing to the immune system and helpful for treating chronic infections and recovering from acute illness or trauma.

How to Use Ashwagandha

Ashwagandha is a very popular plant for many great reasons. This botanical can be enjoyed in tincture, tea, powder, or capsule form. The powder is commonly used in many Ayurvedic food preparations.

Recommended Amounts

DECOCTION: Add 1 teaspoon to 1 tablespoon of dried root (cut and sifted) per cup of water. Simmer for 10 minutes, then steep for 30 minutes. Drink ½ cup, 3 times a day.

DRIED ROOT: 3 to 6 grams per day

STANDARDIZED EXTRACT (1.5% WITHANOLIDES): 300 to 600 milligrams per day

TINCTURE (1:2): 3 to 5 milliliters, 2 or 3 times per day

Cautions and Considerations

Ashwagandha is a nightshade herb and therefore is not recommended for people with nightshade sensitivities, as this may worsen inflammatory conditions in the body such as joint pain, skin rashes, and autoimmune diseases. (Common nightshade vegetables include potatoes, tomatoes, eggplant, and bell peppers.)

Recipes

Ashwagandha is traditionally mixed with ghee or milk to increase absorption. It can be used alone or mixed with other herbs, added to smoothies or made into delicious teas.

Ashwagandha Ghee

MAKES 2 CUPS | Prep time: 2 minutes | Cook time: 10 minutes

Ghee has been used in Ayurvedic medicine for centuries. Ghee, just like ashwagandha, is considered to be a rasayana, a healing food for the body and mind. It stimulates digestive enzymes, optimizes nutrient absorption, and increases the bioavailability of herbs. The combination of ashwagandha and ghee serves as a delicious medicinal food that is nourishing and supportive to the body as a whole.

1 pound organic unsalted butter (ideally grass-fed), diced
½ cup ashwagandha powder

Honey, ginger, or other herbs or spices (optional)

1. In a saucepan, melt the butter over low heat. As the butter starts to melt, mix in the ashwagandha. Melting the butter will separate it into three layers. The milk solids will sink to the bottom of the pan, the clarified butter will be in the middle, and foam will sit on top.

2. Bring the butter to a simmer for 4 to 5 minutes, or until the middle layer is fragrant and golden. The milk solids at the bottom of the pan will also begin to brown. Remove from heat and, using a spoon or strainer, skim off the top layer of foam. Allow the butter to settle for a minute, then carefully pour the golden central layer through a fine-mesh strainer into a glass mason jar. Add honey, ginger, or other herbs or spices for added flavor. Allow the ghee to set for 1 day at room temperature. Store at room temperature for several weeks.

3. To use medicinally, take 1 tablespoon per day. Spread the ghee on toast or dinner rolls, mix into smoothies, or drink in warm milk or tea. You can also eat the ghee by itself or cook it into other foods.

Ashwagandha Moon Milk

SERVES 1 | Prep time: 1 minute | Cook time: 5 minutes

One traditional use of ashwagandha in Ayurvedic medicine is as a sleep tonic. The powdered herb is mixed with warm milk or ghee and combined with cardamom, nutmeg, or other herbs and spices. Nutmeg also has a long history of use in Ayurvedic medicine for its sleep-promoting benefits.

1 cup organic cow's milk, coconut milk, or almond milk

½ teaspoon ashwagandha powder

½ teaspoon curcumin powder (for added stress relief and anti-inflammatory effects) (optional)

Dash ground nutmeg

In a small saucepan, combine the milk, ashwagandha, curcumin (if using), and nutmeg over medium heat. Whisk together until blended well. Heat for 3 to 5 minutes until hot. Pour into a mug and enjoy.

VARIATION: If you're not a milk drinker, you can make this recipe with water and add 4 ounces of tart cherry juice with the ashwagandha power. Tart cherry juice is high in melatonin and is helpful for sleep promotion. It will also sweeten up the bitter taste of the ashwagandha. Serve the drink warm or cold.

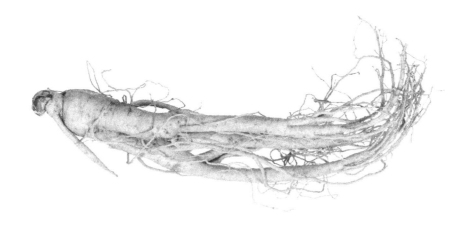

Asian Ginseng

LATIN NAME: *Panax ginseng*

Asian ginseng has been used for thousands of years in Traditional Chinese Medicine (TCM). Its Latin name, *Panax ginseng*, is derived from the Greek word *panacea*, which means "cure all." In TCM, it is considered an herb that tonifies the qi (energy life force) and calms the shen (mind). It is clinically used to replenish the life force, increase the production of body fluids, and promote health and longevity.

Asian ginseng is a traditional treatment for the nervous system. It is a soothing nervine and has often been taken by individuals with nervousness and hysteria. Asian ginseng also has antidepressant activity and is especially helpful to individuals with low mood, weakness, and depletion. It is effective at improving memory and protecting against neurodegeneration as well.

Asian ginseng is native to northeastern China, Korea, and Russia. It is a perennial plant that grows up to two feet tall. Harvesting of Asian ginseng root takes at least six years. There are about six different species of the plant. Asian ginseng is available for purchase in red or white variants. All ginsengs are white when peeled, but when steamed, the root turns red. This steaming process makes the root more stimulating and warming. Asian ginseng is considered the strongest of all the ginsengs.

Asian Ginseng at a Glance

HELPFUL PARTS: root

ADDITIONAL NAMES: Chinese or Korean ginseng, ginseng, Ren Shen

COMMON PREPARATIONS: capsules, decoction, dried root/crude plant, tincture

ENERGETICS AND TASTE: bitter, moist, sweet, warm. Taken in small doses, it is tridoshic (balancing to the three Ayurvedic states).

MEDICINAL PROPERTIES: adaptogenic, cardioprotective, circulation enhancer, hepatoprotective, hypoglycemic/insulin sensitizing, hypolipidemic, immune-modulating, stimulant, tonic, tumor inhibitor

IDEAL FOR ADDRESSING: adrenal fatigue, athletic performance, brain fog and poor memory, cancer prevention and treatment, cardiovascular function, erectile dysfunction and male infertility, immunity, peak performance, weakness/debility

Benefits

ENERGY AND VITALITY: Asian ginseng is especially useful for individuals who have a decreased ability to handle stress and feel mentally, emotionally, and physically exhausted. These states of exhaustion are commonly found in people with extreme adrenal fatigue. Asian ginseng can increase a person's ability to handle stress and improve their vitality and stamina. It is most frequently recommended for use by the elderly and individuals with low vitality, deficiencies, or poor circulation.

Asian ginseng is unique in its ability to provide an immediate boost of energy while also acting to tonify and restore energy and strength to the body.

SEXUAL FUNCTION: One of the first-known uses of Asian ginseng was for treating erectile dysfunction and enhancing male sexual vitality. It is still commonly used in those ways today. It has also been shown to be helpful in treating male infertility. A double-blind study published in the *Chinese Journal of Integrative Medicine* in 2016 showed that supplementation of varicocelectomy surgery with 1½ grams of Asian ginseng per day for a three-month period improved sperm count and motility in infertile men.

IMMUNITY: Asian ginseng is useful for treating chronic conditions and infections where there is a decreased resistance to illness. It improves immunity by increasing white blood cell count and enhancing antibody production. It also increases production of macrophages, which identify and destroy foreign pathogens; natural killer cells, which kill viruses and tumor cells; and interferons, which play a role in cell signaling and immune response. Asian ginseng even acts as an immune modulator, which can be helpful for individuals with allergies and asthma.

It is an excellent adjunctive cancer therapy when used in combination with chemotherapy. It enhances the body's resistance to chemotherapeutic drugs, increases white blood cell count, and improves immune function in cancer patients.

ENHANCED PERFORMANCE: Asian ginseng was the first adaptogen studied and used in Russia. It is well-known for its ability to improve mental and physical stamina and performance. Asian ginseng has also been shown to increase oxygen availability and fatty acid metabolism in the muscles, boosting athletic endurance. It reduces inflammation, helps prevent muscle damage from strenuous exercise, and assists muscle recovery. All of these qualities make it an ideal plant medicine for professional athletes. Asian ginseng improves mental and cognitive functioning and enhances memory, making it useful for students who desire to increase their performance and accuracy when taking tests.

CARDIOVASCULAR FUNCTION AND BLOOD SUGAR REGULATION: Asian ginseng is a circulatory stimulant. It increases circulation and decreases the risk of blood clotting. A clinical study published in *Pharmacological Research* in 2003 suggested it can effectively decrease cholesterol and triglyceride levels and improve cardiac function. In cases of cardiac ischemia, Asian ginseng has been shown to restore coronary blood flow to normal levels. Its anti-inflammatory and antioxidant properties also provide protection to the heart and blood vessels. It can be helpful to individuals with mild hypertension, elevated cholesterol, circulation issues, erectile dysfunction, Raynaud's phenomenon, and congestive heart conditions.

Asian ginseng has hypoglycemic effects and decreases insulin sensitivity. It can be used as an adjunctive treatment by individuals with metabolic syndrome, insulin resistance, and diabetes.

How to Use Asian Ginseng

Asian ginseng has been used in Chinese medicinal cooking for many centuries. The root can be eaten raw or cooked into stews and broths. Asian ginseng is also commonly consumed in tincture, capsule, powder, or tea form.

Recommended Amounts

CAPSULES (POWDERED HERB): 400 to 500 milligrams, 2 or 3 times per day

CRUDE PLANT: 5 to 10 grams per day

DECOCTION: Add 1 teaspoon to 1 tablespoon of dried root (cut and sifted) to 1 to 1½ cups of water. Simmer for 30 minutes, then steep for an additional half hour. Drink ½ cup, 2 to 3 times per day.

TINCTURE (1:2): 1 to 3 milliliters, 2 or 3 times per day

TINCTURE (1:5): 2 to 5 milliliters, 2 or 3 times per day

Cautions and Considerations

Overstimulation may occur in large doses or in sensitive individuals, especially if combined with caffeine or other stimulants. Asian ginseng should be avoided by people who are taking MAO inhibitors, as the combination can increase the risk of manic symptoms.

Asian ginseng can inhibit platelet aggregation and therefore should not be taken with warfarin, a common blood-thinning medication (unless closely monitored by a physician). Pay close attention to any signs of potential hemorrhagic concerns, such as heavy menstrual bleeding or frequent nosebleeds.

Recipes

The whole Asian ginseng root can be cooked into stews and broths. Try adding it to your favorite beef stew, pork soup, or bone broth for a nourishing and energizing boost.

Restorative Bone Broth

MAKES 16 CUPS | Prep time: 10 minutes |

Cook time: 24 hours in slow cooker, 4 to 8 hours on stove top

Bone broth is a soup that is rich in minerals, proteins, and nutrients needed to heal body tissues. It is particularly nourishing for people who are healing from surgery or have inflammatory and digestive concerns. It is recommended to use organic bones and vegetables. Bone broth can be drunk as a warm beverage or used in soups or as a braising liquid.

1 gallon water
2 to 4 pounds meat or
    poultry bones
1 or 2 large onions,
    coarsely chopped
2 carrots, coarsely chopped
3 celery stalks, coarsely chopped

1 bunch parsley
1 or 2 Asian ginseng roots
2 ounces dried astragalus root
4 tablespoons apple cider vinegar
2 or 3 garlic cloves,
    lightly smashed
1 teaspoon salt

1. In a large slow cooker, combine the water, bones, onions, carrots, celery, parsley, ginseng, astragalus, vinegar, garlic, and salt and cook on low heat for 12 to 24 hours. The longer it cooks, the more nutrients are infused into the broth.
2. Strain the stock through a fine-mesh strainer and serve warm. Enjoy 1 to 2 (1-cup) servings per day. Store in an airtight container in the refrigerator for up to 5 days, or freeze for up to 6 months.

VARIATION: Bone broth can also be made on the stove top in a large stockpot. Add all the ingredients, cover, and simmer for 4 to 8 hours.

Male Sexual Tonic

MAKES 120 MILLILITERS (4 OUNCES) |
Prep time: 2 minutes

This tonic can be used to enhance sexual performance, improve fertility, increase sex drive, and optimize energy and stamina.

45 milliliters Asian ginseng (1:2)   35 milliliters rhodiola (1:4)
40 milliliters ashwagandha (1:2)

1. Using a funnel, measure the Asian ginseng, ashwagandha, and rhodiola tinctures in a graduated cylinder, then transfer to a 4-ounce glass bottle.
2. Take a dose of 2 milliliters 2 to 3 times per day.

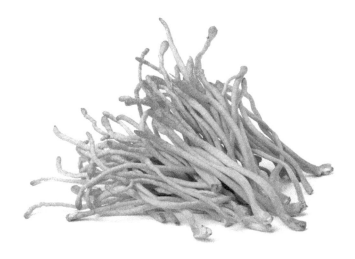

Cordyceps

LATIN NAMES: *Cordyceps sinensis, Cordyceps militaris*

Cordyceps is another adaptogen that has been used in China for thousands of years. Because it was traditionally scarce and so highly valued, it was exclusively reserved for use by the emperor's family. It was prepared by stuffing the fungi in a duck before cooking. The family would then eat this delicacy for 8 to 10 days as a restorative tonic.

Cordyceps is a fungus that grows wild in the Himalayan foothills of Tibet and Bhutan. It is a parasitic fungus that infects and devours the caterpillar larvae of ghost moths. It then grows a stalk and fruiting body, which releases more spores for reproduction. Due to the nature of its development, the Chinese would commonly refer to cordyceps as "winter worm, summer grass."

Cordyceps sinensis is the wild, less common form of cordyceps that still grows on caterpillars. *Cordyceps militaris* is the cultivated form used in commercial production that can be grown on rice extract. *Cordyceps militaris* provides the same nutrients and similar effects as *Cordyceps sinensis* and is a sustainable source that doesn't threaten the wild cordyceps species.

Cordyceps at a Glance

HELPFUL PARTS: fungus, mycelial extract

ADDITIONAL NAMES: caterpillar mushroom, Chinese caterpillar fungus, winter worm, summer grass

COMMON PREPARATIONS: capsules, decoction, edible, extract, powder, tincture

ENERGETICS AND TASTE: moist, slightly acrid, sweet, warm

MEDICINAL PROPERTIES: adaptogenic, antioxidant, antitumor, endocrine-modulating, hypolipidemic, immune-modulating, kidney protective, liver protective

IDEAL FOR ADDRESSING: allergies, asthma, athletic performance, autoimmune conditions, fatigue, frequent urination, infertility, kidney dis-ease

Benefits

ENERGY AND STAMINA: Cordyceps is most notable for its energizing effects and ability to reduce fatigue. This fungus is restorative, regenerative, and nourishing to the body. Cordyceps boosts energy by increasing red blood cell count, helping the heart pump more effectively, and improving protein metabolism.

The beta glucans found in cordyceps drive oxygenation and ATP production, increasing cellular energy and reducing oxidative stress. These qualities make cordyceps an ideal medicinal food for athletes to help protect against overtraining. Cordyceps gained popular attention in 1993 when the coach of several Chinese athletes who broke world records in track and field events attributed much of their success to the use of cordyceps.

IMMUNITY: Cordyceps boosts immune function by increasing the activity of macrophages and natural killer cells (two types of white blood cells) to fight off and kill pathogens. This fungus also increases levels of immune-signaling cytokines interleukin-2 and interferon gamma. Interleukin-2 regulates the activity of white blood cells, and interferon gamma regulates other cytokine and immune cell function. According to a study published in *Functional Foods* in 2017, cordyceps may have antibacterial properties against many pathogenic bacteria strains.

Cordyceps helps prevent chemotherapy-induced immune suppression and improves recovery. It is reported to possess potent cytotoxic activity and has been shown to reduce tumor size in certain cancers (Lim et al, 2009).

These medicinal fungi regulate immune function and reduce allergic and histamine responses. They are effective supplemental medicines for treating allergies, asthma, and autoimmune conditions.

KIDNEY HEALTH: In Chinese medicine, cordyceps is used as a kidney tonic for both excess and deficient conditions. In TCM, the kidneys store the essence of life, the "jing," and also control fluid metabolism, bone health, and healthy sexual functioning. Kidney imbalances often manifest in the ear, and tinnitus can be a common manifestation of kidney essence deficiency. Cordyceps is one of the medicines commonly used to treat kidney imbalances of frequent urination, infertility, erectile dysfunction, loss of libido, tinnitus, and fatigue.

Cordyceps is widely used in TCM for the treatment of chronic kidney dis-ease. It helps improve and preserve kidney function. Its antioxidant properties also provide protection to kidney cells. Cordyceps in conjunction with conventional Western medicine has been shown to improve kidney function in cases of chronic kidney dis-ease and kidney failure. Cordyceps is also often used clinically in the treatment of inflammatory, autoimmune, or degenerative kidney conditions.

LIVER HEALTH: Cordyceps is known to be protective to the liver. In a study published in *Zhongguo Zhong Yao Za Zhi* in 1990, 33 patients with chronic hepatitis B infection showed improved liver function using cordyceps treatment. These individuals displayed increased liver function, plasma albumin levels, and protein metabolism. Similar studies have also shown improvements in liver function in patients with chronic hepatitis B and C infections, and cirrhosis of the liver.

How to Use Cordyceps

Cordyceps is well-known for its restorative and regenerative qualities. This tonic can be taken in the morning, during the day, or at night. It is an endocrine modulator and supports healthy immune function and cell growth. Cordyceps can be enjoyed as a tincture, tea, powder, or capsule, or eaten whole as a delicious medicinal food.

Recommended Amounts

CAPSULES (ETHANOL-EXTRACTED): 1.5 grams per day

EXTRACT: 3 to 9 grams per day

EDIBLE (COOKED WHOLE FUNGUS): 1 cup, 1 or 2 times per day

TINCTURE (1:4, 1:5): 1 to 2 milliliters, 2 or 3 times per day

DECOCTION: Add ¼ to ½ teaspoon of crushed fungi or mycelial powder to 1¼ cups of water. Simmer for 15 minutes, then steep for 1 hour. Drink 1 to 2 cups per day.

Cautions and Considerations

Cordyceps is very safe, and side effects are rare. Side effects can include nausea and transient diarrhea.

Cordyceps is safe to use during pregnancy and breastfeeding. However, raw consumption of these fungi should be avoided. For consumption, they should be washed thoroughly and then cooked.

Recipe

Cordyceps are not only immune-modulating but also high in many nutrients and protein. Cooking the fungus allows for the best nutrient and protein absorption. Cordyceps can be added to soups or stews or combined with veggies or eggs.

Immunity Soup

SERVES 6 | Prep time: 5 minutes, plus 30 minutes soak time | Cook time: 1 hour

This soup is strengthening to the immune system and body as a whole. It can be used as a preventive immune tonic during the cold and flu season or as a treatment for chronic viral, tick-borne, or other infections. This soup can also be used as a preventive or medicinal food in cancer patients and is especially beneficial for those undergoing or recovering from chemotherapy or radiation treatments.

2 to 3 ounces dried astragalus root

6 ounces cordyceps

6 ounces black reishi mushrooms, sliced

2 cups bone broth, vegetable broth, or chicken stock

1 cup water

1 ounce fresh ginger, peeled and sliced

2 garlic cloves, chopped

1 head bok choy, sliced

1½ cups chopped organic kale or spinach

1 large organic onion, chopped

1. Soak the astragalus root in water for 30 minutes, then drain.
2. Trim the bottom part off of the cordyceps and black reishi mushrooms (but not the whole stem) and discard. Slice the remaining caps and stems. (If you do not have fresh mushrooms, you can use dried mushrooms. To use, soak them in 2 cups of boiling water, covered, for 30 minutes. Drain the rehydrated mushrooms and chop. Save the strained mushroom broth for other use, or discard.)
3. In a pot, combine the astragalus root, mushrooms, broth, water, ginger, and garlic. Simmer for 45 minutes.
4. Add the bok choy, kale, and onion. Simmer for another 10 to 15 minutes, until the vegetables are tender.
5. Remove from heat and remove astragalus root.
6. Serve warm. Enjoy 1 to 2 servings per day.

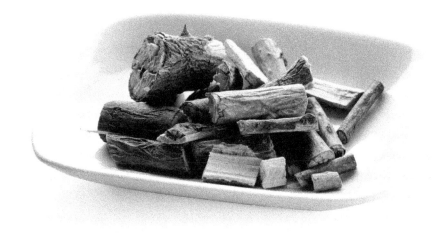

Eleuthero

LATIN NAME: *Eleutherococcus senticosus*

Eleuthero, also known as Siberian ginseng, is an adrenal adaptogen. It helps offset the negative effects of chronic stress by protecting the body from various chemical and environmental stressors. It is less stimulating than Asian ginseng (see page 47), and its uses can be more widely applied. Eleuthero is a great herb for individuals with general fatigue and weakness, decreased physical and mental capacity, lowered immunity, depressed mood, and difficulty concentrating.

Eleuthero is one of the most-studied adaptogenic herbs. In TCM, it is considered to be strengthening and nourishing to the qi. It is used to strengthen the spleen, nourish the kidneys, and reduce blood stagnation.

Eleuthero is more neutral in energetics and action than Asian ginseng (see page 47) and can therefore be more generally applied to the average person. It is a great everyday herb for anyone who is overstressed, overworked, sleep-deprived, and fatigued, such as caretakers, night shift workers, and students. It is best used over the long term for enhancing stamina in those with chronic stress or dis-ease. It is also a favorite plant among athletes for its effectiveness at enhancing endurance and reducing recovery time.

Eleuthero at a Glance

HELPFUL PARTS: root, stem bark

ADDITIONAL NAMES: *Acanthopanax senticosus*, Siberian ginseng

COMMON PREPARATIONS: capsules, decoction, powder, solid extract, tincture

ENERGETICS AND TASTE: neutral to slightly warm, slightly bitter, sweet

MEDICINAL PROPERTIES: adaptogenic, antioxidant, chemoprotective, hypolipidemic, immune-modulating

IDEAL FOR ADDRESSING: athletic performance, chronic stress, fatigue, high cholesterol, recovery from surgery, immune function

Benefits

MENTAL AND PHYSICAL PERFORMANCE: Chronic stress can cause mental and physical fatigue. Eleuthero is a great herb for combating those effects. It has been shown to have a positive influence on mental work capacity and performance, increasing alertness and improving cognitive function. Both professional and amateur athletes commonly use eleuthero for its anti-fatigue qualities and to enhance physical endurance and stamina. It increases cellular energy production and reduces lactic acid buildup in muscles, decreasing muscle soreness and improving recovery time. It can also help prevent immune depletion from overtraining.

IMMUNE FUNCTION: Eleuthero is an immune tonic and regulator. Repeated studies have shown that regular use of this plant improves immunity and decreases sick days of workers.

Eleuthero increases CD4 T-lymphocyte immune cell count and activity. CD4 cells are typically low in number in individuals with HIV, chronic viral infections, or cancer. Eleuthero should be considered as a safe and effective supplemental treatment option for patients with those conditions.

Eleuthero works well as an adjunctive chemotherapy treatment. It protects against immune suppression and white blood cell decrease. It has been shown to extend survival time in cancer patients, improve general health, and decrease side effects from chemotherapy and radiation.

RECOVERY: Research on eleuthero has found that this plant can increase resistance to stressors such as heat, cold, trauma, chemicals, surgery, radiation, toxins, and pathogens. It promotes healing and reduces recovery time when used after surgery or other traumas. It helps the body build back its resilience and ability to respond to stress.

Eleuthero is a powerful antioxidant and reduces the damage to cells caused by radiation, chemotherapy drugs, or chemical carcinogens. It also helps protect against and reduce damage from heavy metals and pesticides.

CARDIOVASCULAR HEALTH: Clinical studies have shown that eleuthero lowers LDL cholesterol and triglyceride levels and can help relieve symptoms of angina. According to the Proceedings of the Second International Symposium on Eleutherococcus, animal studies have shown that eleuthero also increases mitochondria count and improves oxygenation and repair in cardiac muscle. It is helpful for normalizing blood pressure in both hypotensive and hyper-tensive conditions. It is most useful for preventing stress-induced cardiovascular dis-ease.

How to Use Eleuthero

Eleuthero can be enjoyed in tincture, solid extract, tea, capsule, or powder form.

Recommended Amounts

CAPSULES (DRIED HERB): 2 to 4 grams per day

SOLID EXTRACT (4:1): ¼ teaspoon, 2 times per day

ELEUTHEROSIDE B AND E EXTRACT: 200 to 400 milligrams per day

TINCTURE (1:2): 2 to 3 milliliters, 2 or 3 times per day

TINCTURE (1:4, 1:5): 3 to 5 milliliters, 2 or 3 times per day

DECOCTION: Add 1 teaspoon to 1 tablespoon of dried root to 1½ cups of water. Simmer for 20 to 30 minutes, then steep for 1 hour. Drink 2 to 3 cups per day.

Cautions and Considerations

Eleuthero is a very safe herb, and no side effects have been reported in healthy individuals.

Eleuthero has been shown to enhance the effectiveness of some antibiotics.

Use caution when also taking digoxin drugs, as one case of elevated serum digoxin levels with the concurrent use of eleuthero has been reported.

Pregnancy Category B1: There is no evidence of increased frequency of malformation or other harmful effects on the fetus from limited use of eleuthero in women. There is also no evidence of increased fetal damage in animal studies.

Lactation Category C: Eleuthero is compatible with breastfeeding.

Recipe

Eleuthero powder can be easily added to smoothies, protein shakes, or other food recipes as a powerhouse ingredient.

Eleuthero Energy Balls

MAKES 20 BALLS | Prep time: 10 minutes, plus 30 minutes chill time

These eleuthero energy balls are packed with protein, omega-3 fatty acids, and adaptogenic power. This combo serves as a quick way to boost your energy, fuel your body, and support your overall health.

1 cup organic oats
½ cup organic peanut butter,
　almond butter, or other
　nut butter

½ cup ground flaxseed
　(preferable to grind fresh
　before use)
½ cup eleuthero powder
3 to 5 tablespoons honey
2 tablespoons chia seeds

1. In a bowl, combine the oats, nut butter, flaxseed, eleuthero honey, and chia seeds. Cover and chill dough in the refrigerator for 30 minutes.
2. Remove the dough from the refrigerator and roll into 1-inch round balls.
3. Enjoy 2 energy balls per serving 1 to 3 times per day as a healthy breakfast snack, on the go, or as an afternoon pick-me-up. Store in the refrigerator for up to a week.

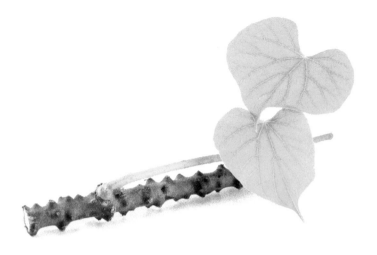

Guduchi

LATIN NAME: *Tinospora cordifolia*

Guduchi is another plant that is classified as a rasayana in Ayurvedic medicine. It is a large climbing deciduous plant that grows in the tropical areas of India and China. The name guduchi means "one which protects the entire body."

Guduchi has been used for centuries in traditional Ayurvedic medicine and folk medicine. In Ayurvedic medicine, it is considered to be one of the best herbs for fixing Pitta and Vata imbalances. It is unique in its warming energetics and ability to clear excess heat (or Pitta) from the body.

Guduchi is gentle in action and is a great herb for people who are very sensitive to or have heightened reactions to medications and herbs. It supports energy, improves the body's resistance to illness, and promotes overall health and longevity.

Guduchi at a Glance

HELPFUL PARTS: root, stem

ADDITIONAL NAMES: amrita, giloe, heart-leaved moonseed, Indian tinospora, kuan jin teng

COMMON PREPARATIONS: decoction, extract, powder, tincture

ENERGETICS AND TASTE: bitter, dry, warm

MEDICINAL PROPERTIES: adaptogenic, anti-allergic, anti-arthritic, anti-inflammatory, antibacterial, antioxidant, antipyretic, antitumor, bone protective, immune-modulating, diuretic, hepatoprotective

IDEAL FOR ADDRESSING: allergies, arthritis, asthma, cancer, fatigue, fevers, gout, hepatitis, jaundice, stress

Benefits

ASTHMA AND ALLERGY MANAGEMENT: Guduchi has been commonly used in Ayurvedic medicine to treat asthma, allergies, and chronic coughs. In one clinical study published in the *Journal of Ethnopharmacology*, regular consumption of guduchi for eight weeks was connected to significant improvement in all symptoms of allergic rhinitis. In this study, 83 percent of people reported a complete resolution of sneezing, 71 percent reported relief from nasal itching, 69 percent reported resolution of nasal discharge, and 61 percent reported improvement of nasal obstruction.

Other studies have shown that guduchi reduces allergic histamine-induced bronchospasms and promotes bronchodilation of the lungs, making it especially effective for treating allergy-induced asthmatic conditions.

IMMUNE HEALTH: Modern studies have shown that guduchi has significant fever-reducing activity, along with antibacterial activity against *Escherichia coli*, *Salmonella* Typhi, *Staphylococcus aureus*, *Proteus vulgaris*, and *Serratia marcescens*. These studies have confirmed the historical uses of this plant in treating fevers and various infections.

This botanical has been found to up-regulate the antitumor effects of tumor-associated macrophages and effectively kill various types of cancer cells in in vitro and mouse studies. Some studies on mice have also shown that guduchi can inhibit carcinogenesis (cancer formation) and metastasis (spread of cancer). Guduchi also helps protect against bone marrow suppression from chemotherapy medications.

ARTHRITIS MANAGEMENT: Guduchi has traditionally been used to treat various arthritic conditions. The anti-inflammatory and immune-modulating actions of this plant benefit individuals with rheumatoid arthritis, which is an autoimmune condition that attacks the joints. Guduchi has been found to have similar effects to non-steroidal anti-inflammatory drugs. It also has bone-building effects, and studies combining guduchi and ginger have found the treatment may lead to pain reduction and improvements in patients with osteo-arthritis. Guduchi increases urinary excretion of uric acid, making it a useful plant for treating gout and gouty arthritis.

LIVER HEALTH: Various studies have shown that guduchi is a powerful liver protectant. It has been found to normalize liver enzyme function, increase liver immune cell function, and stimulate liver cell regeneration. It has also been found to protect the liver against damage from various chemicals and pharmaceuticals. In vitro studies suggest it can quickly inactivate hepatitis B and E surface antigens, and it is often used in the treatment of both acute and chronic hepatitis infections. It is also commonly used to treat jaundice and promote healthy liver function and detoxification.

How to Use Guduchi

The traditional method of consuming guduchi is in decoction form. It can also be enjoyed in tincture, powder, or extract form.

Recommended Amounts

EXTRACT (5:1): 1 gram mixed in water, 1 to 3 times per day

TINCTURE (1:5): 1 to 2 milliliters, 3 times per day

DECOCTION: Add 1 teaspoon of dried herb to 1 cup of water. Simmer for 10 to 15 minutes, then steep for 30 minutes. Drink 4 ounces 2 or 3 times per day.

Cautions and Considerations

Large doses of guduchi can cause constipation.

Recipes

The traditional way to consume guduchi is as a powder made from the stems of the plant. This powder is mixed in warm water with honey to sweeten the bitter taste. In Ayurvedic medicine, this form of the plant is called guduchi kashayam.

Arthritis Relief Tea

MAKES 2 (8-OUNCE) SERVINGS | Prep time: 1 minute | Cook time: 30 minutes

This tea is beneficial for treating osteoarthritis, rheumatoid arthritis, and arthritis caused by gout. It is anti-inflammatory and analgesic and supports healthy bone growth. Feel free to double the ingredients to increase the serving size. This drink can also be used to support healthy blood sugar levels.

2 guduchi stems

1 inch fresh turmeric root

2 cups water

Dash freshly ground black pepper

1 teaspoon raw honey

1. Peel the guduchi and chop into small pieces. Slice the turmeric thinly.
2. In a small saucepan, combine the water, guduchi, and turmeric. Bring to a boil, then simmer for 30 minutes. Remove from heat and strain, reserving the liquid. Discard the remaining root and stems. Add a dash of pepper to increase turmeric absorption.
3. Serve warm as a tea, and add a teaspoon of honey per serving to sweeten. Drink 2 cups daily.

Immunity Juice

MAKES 3 CUPS | Prep time: 5 minutes

Enjoy this delicious immune-boosting juice when you are sick or as a preventive measure. It's also great for lowering blood sugar, treating allergies, improving digestion, and boosting energy.

2 or 3 guduchi stems

2 cups distilled water

1 cup fresh organic spinach

½ inch fresh ginger, peeled and thinly sliced or grated

8 to 10 fresh holy basil leaves

1 teaspoon cordyceps powder (~1.5 grams)

Juice of 1 lemon

1. Peel the guduchi and chop into small pieces.
2. Put the guduchi, water, spinach, ginger, holy basil, and cordyceps into the blender. Cut the lemon in half and squeeze the juice into the blender. Blend until a smooth liquid is formed.
3. Enjoy as a delicious immune-boosting juice. For maintenance and prevention, drink 1 cup per day. To boost the immune system while sick, drink 2 to 3 cups per day.

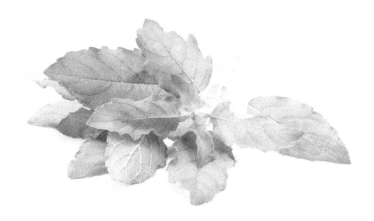

Holy Basil

LATIN NAME: *Ocimum sanctum*

Holy basil is a plant native to India and Southeast Asia. It has a long history of use in Ayurvedic medicine and has traditionally been considered one of India's most powerful plants. Holy basil is often referred to as "The Incomparable One," "The Queen of Herbs," and the "Mother Medicine of Nature."

Holy basil is considered to be an "elixir of life." It is physically, emotionally, cognitively, and spiritually healing. In Ayurvedic medicine, it is considered to be a rasayana and tridoshic, bringing balance to all three of the Ayurvedic constitutions: Pitta, Kapha, and Vata. Regular use of this herb is also believed to balance the chakras of the body.

Holy basil is the most sacred plant in Hinduism. It is commonly found in households and used in daily prayers to achieve spiritual purity, health, and wellness. It is often cultivated in temples and used in religious ceremonies as well. Some Hindu and Greek Orthodox churches include this medicinal plant in holy water.

Holy Basil at a Glance

HELPFUL PARTS: plant

ADDITIONAL NAMES: sacred basil, tulsi

COMMON PREPARATIONS: capsules, tea, tincture

ENERGETICS AND TASTE: pungent, sweet, warm

MEDICINAL PROPERTIES: adaptogenic, antidepressant, antioxidant, antiviral, anxiolytic, carminative, diuretic, expectorant, galactagogue, immune-modulating, neuroprotective

IDEAL FOR ADDRESSING: anxiety, blood sugar dysregulation, brain fog, cardiovascular health, depression, detoxification, fatigue, memory issues

Benefits

IMMUNE SUPPORT: Holy basil is an immune amphoteric, meaning it normalizes function of the immune system. It increases counts of natural killer cells and macrophages to fight off pathogens, enhances the immune response, and has antibacterial, antiviral, and antifungal effects. It has historically been used to treat coughs, colds, flus, fevers, sore throats, congestion, wound infections, snakebites, and scorpion stings. It is immune-modulating and anti-inflammatory and decreases histamine reactions. It is a great herb for treating allergies and asthma for these reasons. It contains ursolic acid, which is known to have antitumor effects. It is also protective against radiation- and chemotherapy-induced damage.

OVERALL HEALTH AND WELLNESS: Referred to as the "herb for all reasons," holy basil has widespread benefits for the body as a whole. It has protective effects on the heart, liver, pancreas, and kidneys. It has been demonstrated to lower blood pressure and reduce total cholesterol, LDL cholesterol, and triglyceride levels. It helps decrease and regulate blood sugar levels and improve insulin resistance.

A study done using acetaminophen, which is highly toxic to the liver, showed that holy basil supplementation provided significant hepatoprotective effects. This study also showed that holy basil has synergistic effects with silymarin, the main active constituent of milk thistle, a plant well-known for its protective and regenerative effects on the liver.

MENTAL CLARITY AND MOOD SUPPORT: Holy basil provides many benefits for brain function and mood support. It has been found to improve mental clarity and memory by increasing circulation and oxygenation in the brain. It is thought to bring enlightened thoughts and "brilliance to the mind." It is both calming and uplifting and is an effective antidepressant and anxiolytic herb. It enhances production of our "feel-good" neurotransmitters dopamine and serotonin, which help improve motivation and happiness.

Holy basil is effective at reducing stress and improving sleep. Participants in a six-week study of daily holy basil supplementation reported improvements in the areas of exhaustion, forgetfulness, and sleep.

How to Use Holy Basil

Holy basil is most popularly consumed as a tea. This is the preferred way to nourish the spirit. Tulsi tea can be made with either fresh or dried leaves. The fresh leaves can also be eaten whole. In India, fresh holy basil leaves are commonly consumed in the morning on an empty stomach to boost the immune system. Holy basil is also frequently enjoyed in tincture and capsule form.

Recommended Amounts

CAPSULES (2% URSOLIC ACID, 8.5% EUGENOL): 150 to 300 milligrams, 2 or 3 times per day

EXTRACT: 300 to 2,000 milligrams per day

TINCTURE (1:5): 3 to 5 milliliters, 2 or 3 times per day

TINCTURE (1:2): 2 to 3 milliliters, 3 times per day

TEA: Add 1 or 2 tablespoons of dried leaves (or ½ cup of fresh leaves) to 1 cup of boiling water. Steep for 5 to 10 minutes. Drink 4 ounces 3 times per day.

Cautions and Considerations

Holy basil is thought to have antifertility effects and should therefore be avoided by individuals trying to conceive or undergoing fertility treatment. The effects on pregnant individuals are unclear, and they should also avoid consuming holy basil.

Recipe

Holy basil leaves can be made into various teas, juices, or smoothies or eaten whole. Holy basil combines well with other adaptogenic herbs such as turmeric and ashwagandha.

Tulsi Ka Kadha

MAKES 6 (8-OUNCE) SERVINGS | Prep time: 5 minutes | Cook time: 4 minutes, plus 15 minutes steep time

This is a version of the traditional Indian kadha recipe used to treat colds and flus. Holy basil is well-known for its immune-boosting effects, and when combined with lemongrass and ginger, it makes a potent immunity tea tonic. Lemongrass is commonly known as "fever grass," as it can reduce fevers and alleviate body aches. Lemongrass also has antibacterial and antifungal properties and is very cleansing and detoxifying to the body.

15 fresh holy basil leaves

6 cups water

1 lemongrass stalk, cut into 2-inch pieces

1 inch fresh ginger, peeled and grated

1. Remove the holy basil leaves from the stems, discarding the stems. Soak the leaves in water for 1 to 2 minutes to remove any excess dirt. Drain the leaves and discard the liquid.
2. In a large saucepan, combine the 6 cups of water, holy basil, lemongrass, and ginger and bring to a boil. Boil for 3 to 4 minutes. Remove from heat and steep for 10 to 15 minutes.
3. Strain, reserving the tea, and enjoy warm. Serve 1 cup per day for prevention or up to 2 cups per day to boost the immune system while acutely sick. Store in an airtight container in the refrigerator for several days.

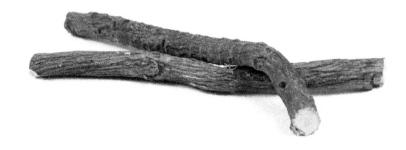

Licorice

LATIN NAME: *Glycyrrhiza glabra, Glycyrrhiza uralensis*

Glycyrrhiza glabra is a plant native to southeastern Europe and southwestern Asia. *Glycyrrhiza uralensis*, commonly known as Chinese licorice, is native to northern China and Russia. It is a perennial that grows 1 to 2 meters high and produces a long, sturdy taproot. This taproot is around 15 centimeters long and divides into smaller rootlets and horizontal woody stolons (plant stems). This deep-rooted, sturdy plant physically matches its strengthening medicinal properties well.

Licorice has been used for thousands of years throughout Europe and Asia as a medicinal plant. It was considered to be one of the best medicines in ancient China for treating various ailments. Shennong's *Materia Medica*, written around 2100 BCE, lists licorice as having life-enhancing properties.

This medicinal plant works on all tissues and has a particular affinity for the gastrointestinal, respiratory, nervous, reproductive, and excretory systems. It has been consumed for centuries to treat sore throats, coughs, constipation and other gastrointestinal issues, and various infections.

Licorice is also a great synergizing herb. I add small amounts to most botanical formulas to help all the herbs work better together. Its sweetness brings the additional benefit of improving taste.

Licorice at a Glance

HELPFUL PARTS: root

ADDITIONAL NAMES: Chinese licorice root, gan cao, sweet grass, sweet root

COMMON PREPARATIONS: capsules, decoction, DGL, dried root, solid extract, tincture, topical salve

ENERGETICS AND TASTE: bitter, cool, moist, sweet

MEDICINAL PROPERTIES: adaptogenic, anti-inflammatory, antioxidant, antiviral, demulcent, hepatoprotective, immune modulating, phytoestrogen

IDEAL FOR ADDRESSING: adrenal fatigue, gastrointestinal issues, immune issues

Benefits

ADRENAL HEALTH: Licorice is unique in its adaptogenic actions and actually works to increase cortisol levels. Licorice root helps prevent the breakdown of cortisol, prolonging its half-life and activity in the body. This effect is attributed to the actions of glycyrrhetinic acid, a primary active constituent of licorice root.

Glycyrrhetinic acid has similar activity to the steroid hormone aldosterone but to a lesser degree. Glycyrrhetinic acid binds to mineralo-corticoid receptors in the adrenal glands and inhibits the breakdown of the primary enzyme that processes cortisol and aldosterone. Because of this, licorice root is a great medicinal herb for people in exhausted states of adrenal fatigue accompanied by low cortisol levels. It can also be a great herb for people with Addison's disease (adrenal insufficiency).

ANTIVIRAL/IMMUNE SUPPORT: Licorice has strong antiviral activity and is often used in the treatment of both acute and chronic viral infections. Licorice root has been shown to stimulate natural killer cell activity and interferon production and inhibit replication of the herpes simplex 1 virus. It is used both internally and topically, along with lemon balm, to treat herpes infections. Licorice has also been found to have antiviral activity against coxsackievirus, influenza, and hepatitis C infections. Its antiviral and liver-protective properties make it an ideal herb for treating hepatitis infections. It is commonly used to treat mononucleosis and chronic fatigue syndrome as well.

Licorice is also great for treating colds, sore throats, coughs, and other acute viral infections. It is recommended specifically for dry and spasmodic coughs and ailments due to its demulcent (soothing), moisturizing, and anti-inflammatory actions.

GASTROINTESTINAL HEALTH: Licorice is very soothing and healing to mucus membranes and is often used to calm inflammation and irritation in the gastrointestinal tract. It can be used to treat peptic ulcer dis-ease, gastrointestinal reflex issues, irritable bowel syndrome, inflammatory bowel disorders, and colitis. The glycyrrhetinic acid component of licorice is typically removed in preparations that are only aimed at healing the gastrointestinal tract. This preparation is called deglycyrrhizinated licorice, or DGL.

Licorice is also a strong protectant for the liver. Its anti-inflammatory and antioxidant properties can reduce liver damage from toxins, pharmaceuticals, and infections.

How to Use Licorice

Licorice can be enjoyed in tincture, tea, solid extract, powder, or capsule form. The dried root can also be cooked into foods. Licorice root adds flavor and enhances the activity of other herbs when used in combination formulas or in cooking. A delicious licorice tea can be a great way to start your morning. Due to its ability to extend the half-life of cortisol, this herb is best taken in the morning and early afternoon to coincide with the body's normal healthy cortisol rhythm.

To avoid the steroidal effects of licorice root, glycyrrhetinic acid components can be removed. Such preparations are commonly used to treat gastrointestinal and urinary inflammation and can be found in powdered or chewable form.

Licorice is also commonly found in topical form, as it is an effective treatment for a variety of skin conditions. Glycyrrhizic acid, the main active constituent of licorice root, is a potent antiviral and has been shown to inactivate herpes simplex virus particles.

Glycyrrhetinic acid, a hydrolytic product of glycyrrhizic acid, has been found to be an effective treatment for atopic dermatitis and psoriasis, exerting similar effects to that of topical hydrocortisone but with a much higher safety profile.

Recommended Amounts

DECOCTION: 1 to 2 teaspoons of dried root (cut and sifted), per 1 cup water. Simmer for 10 to 15 minutes, then steep for 15 minutes. Drink about ½ cup, 2 to 3 times a day.

DGL CAPSULES/CHEWABLE TABLETS: 380 to 760 milligrams, 3 times per day before meals

DGL POWDER: ¼ to ½ teaspoon, 3 times per day before meals

EDIBLE (DRIED ROOT): 1 to 3 grams, 3 times per day

SOLID EXTRACT (4:1): ¼ teaspoon, 2 times per day

TINCTURE (1:5): 3 to 5 milliliters, 2 or 3 times per day

TINCTURE (1:2, 1:3): 1 to 3 milliliters, 2 or 3 times per day

TOPICAL SALVE: apply to affected area several times per day

Cautions and Considerations

Licorice is moistening and can aggravate damp conditions. For example, you should not give high doses of licorice to treat a wet cough. A drying and astringent herb would be better suited for treating this condition.

Long-term ingestion of high doses of licorice can increase reabsorption of sodium and excretion of potassium, creating a pseudoaldosterone (steroid-like) effect. This can cause high blood pressure, low potassium levels, and water retention, which can exacerbate hypertension, congestive heart failure, and renal failure. This herb should be avoided by individuals suffering from these conditions.

Licorice should be avoided in pregnancy. The saponins in licorice inhibit the enzyme that converts androstenedione into testosterone. In high doses, this can decrease testosterone in men. In pregnant women, this may affect male fetal development.

It should not be used in conjunction with cardiac glycoside herbs or medications like digitalis, as it can increase the toxicity of these drugs. It should not be used with potassium-depleting diuretic medications or any medication that depletes potassium levels. Lastly, it should not be used in high doses for prolonged periods of time by young males or individuals with any of the aforementioned risk factors.

Licorice root can help people decrease the dosage of or wean off corticosteroid medications.

Recipe

Licorice root can be cooked into stews and broths to add sweetness and nourishment. This sweetness also makes licorice root an excellent option for teas, on its own or in tea blends. It is often added to tea blends to improve taste and efficacy.

Adrenal Restoration Beef Stew

SERVES 4 | Prep time: 20 minutes | Cook time: 2 hours 10 minutes

This beef stew is great for treating adrenal fatigue, anemia, and compromised immune systems. The bone broth base provides the extra nutritional benefits of amino acids, collagen, and bone marrow, which support gut, joint, and immune health. Licorice root is restorative to the adrenal glands, strengthens the immune system, and provides extra antiviral support, which is beneficial during cold and flu season.

¼ cup all-purpose flour or
gluten-free flour alternative

¼ teaspoon freshly ground
black pepper

1 pound beef stewing meat,
trimmed and cut into
1-inch pieces

1 tablespoon vegetable oil

4 cups bone broth

2 tablespoons red wine vinegar

1 gram dried licorice root, sliced

2 bay leaves

3 medium carrots, cut into
¼-inch rounds

1 large potato, peeled and cut
into ¾-inch cubes

2 celery stalks, cut into
1-inch pieces

1 medium onion, chopped

2 teaspoons sea salt

1 teaspoon garlic powder

1 rosemary sprig

1. In a bowl, combine the flour and pepper, add the beef, and toss to coat well.
2. In a large pot, heat the vegetable oil over medium-high heat. Add the beef and cook for about 10 minutes, stirring as needed, until the meat is browned.
3. Add the bone broth, red wine vinegar, licorice root, and bay leaves. Bring to a boil, then simmer. Cover and cook for 90 minutes until the meat is tender. Add the carrots, potato, celery, onion, salt, garlic powder, and rosemary and cook, covered, for another 30 minutes until the vegetables are tender.
4. Remove the licorice root and bay leaves.
5. Serve warm and enjoy.

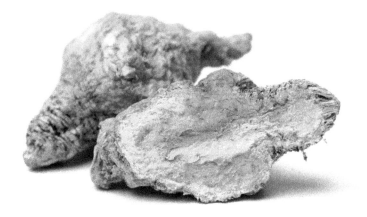

Maca

LATIN NAME: *Lepidium meyenii*

Maca root is a Peruvian plant that grows exclusively in the Andes Mountains at high altitudes. This resilient plant grows at extreme climates consisting of freezing-cold weather, harsh winds, and intense sunlight. Maca is the only crop in the world that is known to thrive in such harsh climates and high elevations. This exposure to extreme environmental factors is what creates the most active constituents of maca, the macamides. Maca cultivation dates back 2000 years and all maca harvesting is done by hand.

Maca is part of the mustard family, and the fresh root looks like a turnip. It has been used for centuries as a nutritious food. The root is rich in phytonutrients, vitamins, minerals, amino acids, and fatty acids. It is high in nutrients that build muscle and nourish the nervous system. Children are thought to thrive both physically and cognitively on a maca-rich diet. Peruvian adults who have consumed this plant since childhood tend to have lower blood pressure, lower body weight, lower incidence of bone fractures, and better health overall than those who did not grow up eating maca.

Maca at a Glance

HELPFUL PARTS: root

ADDITIONAL NAMES: maca-maca, maino

COMMON PREPARATIONS: capsules, decoction, edible, powder, tincture

ENERGETICS AND TASTE: moist, sweet, warm

MEDICINAL PROPERTIES: adaptogenic, mild antidepressant, nutritive tonic, reproductive tonic

IDEAL FOR ADDRESSING: fatigue, infertility, low libido

Benefits

ENERGY, STAMINA, AND VITALITY: One of the first traditional uses of maca was to increase energy and stamina. Inca warriors are believed to have eaten this root before battle to boost their strength and energy. Athletes today consume it to reduce fatigue and enhance stamina and athletic performance. A study done on cyclists for the *Journal of Ethnopharmacology* found that taking maca for 14 consecutive days improved cycling time compared to baseline tests.

Maca has also been shown to optimize brain function and mood, improve cognitive function, and reduce symptoms of anxiety. According to a study published in 2016 in *Evidence-Based Complementary and Alternative Medicine*, maca may increase mitochondrial function and up-regulate proteins that help slow age-related cognitive decline. Many other studies have found that maca is effective at reducing both anxiety and depression. Rat studies published in the *Journal of Medicinal Food* in 2014 discovered that maca's antidepressant effects are related to activation of the dopaminergic and noradrenergic systems. These pathways regulate the production of dopamine and norepinephrine, two neurotransmitters that play an important role in regulating mood, attention, learning, and memory.

FEMALE HEALTH: Maca has a long history of use as a fertility and libido enhancer in women. Maca's adaptogenic effects restore balance in the endocrine system and optimize the function of the reproductive organs and thyroid. Recent studies have shown that maca can increase estrogen and FSH (follicle-stimulating hormone) levels.

Maca is commonly used in the treatment of perimenopausal and menopausal symptoms. Clinical studies have shown it to be effective at reducing hot flashes, night sweats, anxiety, depression, insomnia, fatigue, and low libido. It has an amazing ability to treat all of these menopausal symptoms as a whole instead of just reducing individual symptoms.

MALE HEALTH: Maca has been shown to increase sperm count and motility, libido, and seminal fluid volume. In studies, maca has not appeared to increase levels of testosterone or other sex hormones, so these effects appear to be the result of adaptogenic and endocrine-modulating factors. In high doses, maca has been found to alleviate the common side effect of sexual dysfunction caused by SSRI medications. Maca is also effective at improving sexual desire in men.

How to Use Maca

Maca has a long history of consumption as a functional food and medicine. It is used to enhance energy, vitality, cognitive function, mood, and sexual health. It is most commonly taken in powder or capsule form, but it can also be used as a tincture or tea.

Recommended Amounts

CAPSULES: 500 milligrams, 2 or 3 times per day

POWDER: 1.5 to 5 grams per day

TINCTURE (1:4, 1:5): 4 to 6 milliliters, 3 times per day

DECOCTION: Add 2 teaspoons of powder to 1 cup of water. Simmer for 15 to 20 minutes, then steep for 30 minutes. Drink 8 ounces 3 times per day.

Cautions and Considerations

Maca has no known side effects, contraindications, or drug or herb interactions.

Recipe

The powdered maca herb can be used to make teas and other beverages.

Women's Vitality Smoothie

MAKES 1 (24-OUNCE) SMOOTHIE | Prep time: 2 minutes

This smoothie is great for supporting women's endocrine health. It can be used to treat hormonal imbalances, menopausal symptoms, low libido, and fatigue as well as to enhance fertility.

1 cup frozen organic berries
 of choice
1 cup water
½ cup frozen organic spinach

1 to 2 scoops protein powder
 of choice
1 tablespoon almond butter
1 teaspoon shatavari powder
1 teaspoon maca powder

Put the berries, water, spinach, protein powder, almond butter, shatavari, and maca into a blender and process until smooth. Serve immediately.

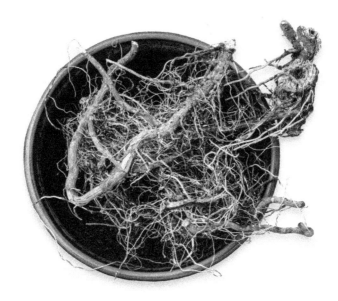

Rhaponticum

LATIN NAME: *Rhaponticum carthamoides*

Rhaponticum is a perennial plant native to Siberia. It was originally used to help people survive the harsh winter climates and as a plant tonic to help the body wake up from the long winters. It is commonly called maral root because the maral deer in Siberia feed on this plant. These deer have strong musculature, which is believed to be due to rhaponticum.

Rhaponticum has a long history of enhancing physical energy and stamina and improving mood and brain function. It has also been used to enhance male and female sexual health and sex drive.

In traditional Siberian folk medicine, this plant was often coupled with rhodiola. Modern recipes still combine these herbs, and they are often found together in Russian athletic formulas today. Rhaponticum was one of the original adaptogenic plants studied by the Russians, and after 25 years of clinical research, it gained entry into the official Russian Pharmacopoeia.

Its major active constituents are phytoecdysteroids, which enhance protein and muscle synthesis. These are also found in high amounts in spinach and quinoa.

Regular use of rhaponticum promotes muscle building, and it is still widely used by Russian athletes today. Its phytoecdysteroids also increase ATP production and improve the body's adaptability to stress.

Rhaponticum at a Glance

HELPFUL PARTS: root

ADDITIONAL NAMES: maral root

COMMON PREPARATIONS: capsules, decoction, tincture

ENERGETICS AND TASTE: bitter, cool, slightly dry, slightly sweet and resinous

MEDICINAL PROPERTIES: adaptogenic, antidepressant, antioxidant, immune stimulant, nervine

IDEAL FOR ADDRESSING: athletic performance, brain fog, depression, fatigue, sexual health, immune function, stress, work performance

Benefits

ENDURANCE AND RESILIENCE: Rhaponticum supports physical and mental endurance. It helps protect against stress-related issues such as insomnia, poor sleep, foggy thinking, low mood, and exhaustion. It is a stimulating adaptogen that is helpful for improving cognition and depressive states. This plant is often used to increase work efficiency, peak performance, and resilience. Rhaponticum is rejuvenating to the mind and body and is well-known for its energy-boosting effects.

ATHLETIC PERFORMANCE: Rhaponticum has anabolic benefits that increase healthy protein synthesis in muscle tissue and build lean muscle mass. It boosts blood flow and oxygenation to muscles during exercise, helping improve stamina and endurance. It has a long history of use by Russian Olympians to enhance athletic performance. It even helps with muscle recovery from training by encouraging the secretion of lactic acid from muscles.

Rhaponticum supports mitochondrial function and muscle tissue integration and increases energy stores in the muscles. It is especially helpful for preventing catabolic processes commonly associated with stress and can be a useful herb in conditions associated with increased muscle breakdown.

OVERALL HEALTH AND WELLNESS: Rhaponticum is a strong adaptogen that promotes overall health and vitality in the body. It is protective of the liver, increasing energy production and resistance to toxins in liver cells. It is a strong antioxidant and helps reduce free radical damage of bodily tissues. It supports healthy blood sugar levels and promotes healthy fat distribution in the body.

How to Use Rhaponticum

Rhaponticum is a powerful adaptogenic plant that is especially well-known for its muscle-building and performance-enhancing capabilities. This herb can help the average gym-goer and the professional athlete achieve mental and physical peak performance. This plant can be enjoyed in capsule, tincture, or liquid decoction form. To enhance athletic performance, use this plant 30 minutes prior to workouts. Use this plant daily to enhance mental function, boost mood, and increase energy.

Recommended Amounts

STANDARDIZED CAPSULES (5% ECDYSTERONE):
2 capsules, 2 times per day

TINCTURE (1:4, 1:5): 2 to 4 milliliters, 3 times per day

DECOCTION: Add 1 to 2 teaspoons of dried root to 1½ cups of water. Simmer for 15 to 20 minutes, then steep for 40 minutes. Drink 4 ounces 2 times per day.

Cautions and Considerations

Do not use rhaponticum during pregnancy, as it has been shown to induce labor.

Recipe

Rhaponticum is not often found in powder form. Traditional use of this medicine was mostly as a tea. Rhaponticum is not found readily in the United States, but it is a staple adaptogenic plant in Russia.

Happy-Time Tea

**MAKES 3 (4-OUNCE) SERVINGS | Prep time: 1 minute |
Cook time: 15 to 20 minutes, plus 40 minutes steep time**

Consuming this tea in the morning is a great way to start your day. Drinking a second cup in the early afternoon is a great way to fight off that after-lunch fatigue and boost your mood and productivity.

1½ cups water

1 to 2 teaspoons dried rhaponticum root

1. In a small pot, bring the water and rhaponticum to a simmer for 15 to 20 minutes, then steep for 40 minutes.
2. Enjoy 4 ounces of tea 3 times per day.

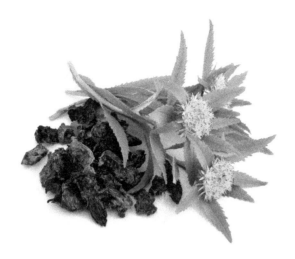

Rhodiola

LATIN NAME: *Rhodiola rosea*

Rhodiola was one of the first adaptogenic plants studied by the USSR, but its historical use dates to long before that. It has a storied history in Siberia, Scandinavia, and Tibet. It was traditionally used in folk medicine to increase physical endurance, productivity, and longevity. Chinese emperors conducted expeditions to Siberia in search of this plant that could boost vitality and reduce susceptibility to illness.

Rhodiola has long been believed to enhance reproductive health and fertility, and it was traditionally given to couples in Siberia as a wedding gift. It was also used by the Vikings of Scandinavia to enhance their physical strength and endurance.

Rhodiola's history piqued the interest of the Soviets, who studied the plant and classified it as an adaptogen. In 1969, it was officially adopted into the Official Russian Pharmacopoeia as an adaptogen, nervous system tonic, and antidepressant.

Rhodiola has become a popular adaptogenic plant today due to its widespread actions and benefits. It is a multipurpose and multisystem medicinal plant, balancing to the endocrine and reproductive systems. It has been found to enhance sexual health and promote fertility, and it boosts cognition, improves mental performance, and encourages general well-being in students. It is also a fantastic herb for athletes or anyone wanting to improve their physical fitness, endurance, and performance. It shortens recovery time from strenuous physical activity and treats immune depletion from overtraining and overwork. It has protective and strengthening effects on the heart and is a powerful antioxidant for the body.

Rhodiola at a Glance

HELPFUL PARTS: root

ADDITIONAL NAMES: Arctic root, golden root, roseroot

COMMON PREPARATIONS: capsules, decoction, powder, tincture

ENERGETICS AND TASTE: astringent, bitter, cool, dry, spicy, sweet

MEDICINAL PROPERTIES: adaptogenic, anti-arrhythmic, antidepressant, antioxidant, antiviral, cardioprotective, immune stimulant, nervous system tonic, neuroprotectant, stimulant

IDEAL FOR ADDRESSING: athletic stamina, brain fog, chronic stress, depression, erectile dysfunction, fatigue, heart conditions, infertility, lowered immunity, peak performance

Benefits

MOOD SUPPORT: Stress and fatigue can be contributing factors to anxiety and depression. Rhodiola is an excellent herb for individuals with these conditions, as it treats these factors.

Rhodiola is beneficial for overall mood support. It has been shown to increase levels of dopamine, norepinephrine, and serotonin. It can be helpful in treating both anxiety and depression, as it provides the dual action of cognitive stimulation and emotional calming. It is best known for its benefits to individuals with depression: A six-week double-blind study linked the use of rhodiola to positive outcomes in individuals with depression, including improvements in sleep, emotional stability, and physical symptoms. But according to a small pilot study published in the *Journal of Alternative and Complementary Medicine* in 2008, 10 people with generalized anxiety disorder also showed improvement with 10 weeks of rhodiola supplementation.

CARDIOVASCULAR HEALTH: Rhodiola has many cardio-protective effects. It can prevent stress-induced cardiac damage and arrhythmias. It improves the strength of the heart and has been shown to reduce recovery time after a heart attack. It also reduces cardio-vascular recovery time after strenuous exercise. It even decreases heart and lung stress at high altitudes and can be taken as a preventive for altitude sickness. It should be considered for consumption by anyone with cardiovascular risk factors, stress-induced heart palpitations, angina, or congestive heart failure.

REPRODUCTIVE HEALTH: Rhodiola is commonly used in the treatment of both male and female infertility. A 1970 study done on women with secondary amenorrhea found that supplementation of 200 milligrams of rhodiola a day for two weeks restored normal menses in 25 of the 40 women. Eleven of those women then went on to become pregnant. Supplementation of 150 to 200 milligrams of rhodiola a day for three months improved erectile function and overall sexual function in 26 of 35 men.

How to Use Rhodiola

Rhodiola can be helpful for the student, the athlete, or the couple trying to conceive. This powerful herb can be enjoyed in tincture, capsule, powder, or tea form. As it is a stimulating adaptogen, it is recommended to avoid using rhodiola after 4 p.m., as it may interfere with sleep if taken in the evening.

Recommended Amounts

CAPSULES (1% ROSAVIIN): 300 to 600 milligrams per day

CAPSULES (2% ROSAVIN): 80 to 300 milligrams per day

TINCTURE (1:4, 1:5): 1 to 3 milliliters, 3 times per day

DECOCTION: Add 1 to 2 teaspoons of dried root to 1¼ cups of water. Simmer for 15 minutes, then steep for 45 minutes. Drink 1 to 2 cups per day.

Cautions and Considerations

Because rhodiola is stimulating to the nervous system and acts to increase serotonin levels, it is contraindicated for people with bipolar disorder, as it can worsen manic states.

High doses of rhodiola may cause irritability and insomnia in some individuals. It is also very drying and may exacerbate dry conditions.

Recipes

Rhodiola root has a strong dry, astringent, bitter taste. It is not as tasty and doesn't cook as well in soups and broths as some of the other root adaptogens. This herb is typically consumed in tincture, capsule, powder, or tea form. In tea form, it is more enjoyable when paired with a sweeter-tasting herb like licorice. In powder form, it can be added to smoothies, protein shakes, and other foods.

Student Study Aid

MAKES 120 MILLILITERS (4 OUNCES) |

Prep time: 2 minutes

This formula is great for students, as it helps improve focus and attention, enhance cognition, and decrease mental fatigue. The addition of gotu kola increases circulation to the brain and boosts memory retention.

40 milliliters rhodiola (1:4)

30 milliliters rhaponticum (1:4)

20 milliliters Asian ginseng (1:2)

30 milliliters gotu kola (1:5)

1. Using a funnel, measure the rhodiola, rhaponticum, Asian ginseng, and gotu kola tinctures in a graduated cylinder, then transfer to a 4-ounce glass bottle.
2. Take a dose of 2 milliliters 3 times per day.

Joyful Tea

MAKES 2 (8-OUNCE) SERVINGS | Prep time: 1 minute |

Cook time: 15 minutes, plus 45 minutes steep time

This tea can be used to boost mood, increase energy, support brain health, and improve libido. It can also be used to treat conditions resulting from hormonal imbalances, such as amenorrhea and symptoms accompanying menopause.

2¼ cups water

1 to 2 teaspoons dried
   rhodiola root

2 teaspoons maca powder

1. In a small pot, combine the water and rhodiola. Simmer for 15 minutes. Add the maca powder, then cover and steep for 45 minutes.
2. Enjoy 2 cups of tea per day.

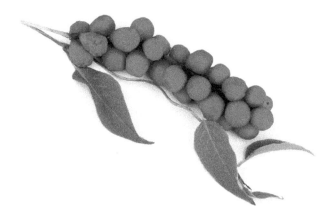

Schisandra

LATIN NAME: *Schisandra chinensis*

Schisandra is a plant native to China. It is an aromatic woody shrub that reaches up to 25 feet in height. It has pink flowers, and its medicinal fruit is a berry. Schisandra is commonly referred to as the "five-flavor fruit" because schisandra berries are believed to contain all five TCM flavors: sweet, salty, spicy, bitter, and sour. Due to this, schisandra is considered a tonic plant that protects and strengthens all five of the yin organs in Chinese medicine: kidneys, liver, heart, lungs, and spleen.

In Chinese folklore, schisandra is believed to calm the heart and the mind. Modern herbalists think of this herb as one that can turn a worrier into a warrior. It is strengthening to the mind and nervous system and works to increase alertness and mental capacity. Like all adaptogens, it supports the body and mind and improves physical and mental performance.

Schisandra at a Glance

HELPFUL PARTS: berry (fruit), seed

ADDITIONAL NAMES: five-flavor fruit, wu wei zi

COMMON PREPARATIONS: capsules, decoction, edible, powder, tincture

ENERGETICS AND TASTE: contains all five flavors (sweet, sour, salty, bitter, pungent), dry, warm

MEDICINAL PROPERTIES: adaptogenic, anti-inflammatory, antioxidant, astringent, immune-modulating, kidney and lung tonic, liver protective, nervine

IDEAL FOR ADDRESSING: anxiety, asthma, depression, detoxification, fatigue, immune deficiency, insomnia, kidney function, liver dis-ease, lung function, palpitations

Benefits

LIVER PROTECTION: Schisandra is one of the best adaptogenic plants for liver health. It is protective of the liver and decreases hepatic damage from toxins, viruses, and free radicals. It is also a potent antioxidant for liver cells and helps produce glutathione (our bodies' most powerful antioxidant and detoxifying agent).

Schisandra increases liver metabolism and enhances both phase 1 and phase 2 liver detoxification pathways. It even accelerates liver repair. It is a useful plant for individuals with chronic hepatitis and liver cirrhosis.

LUNG AND KIDNEY HEALTH: Schisandra is strengthening and tonifying to the lungs and should be considered for consumption by any individual with a constitutional weakness in the lungs. Schisandra is very astringent and drying and is helpful in treating wet coughs. It is also a strong anti-inflammatory and antioxidant, making it especially helpful for treating asthma.

In TCM, schisandra's astringency is also thought to act on the kidneys to treat excessive urination, spontaneous sweating, and night sweats.

NERVOUS SYSTEM FUNCTION: Schisandra is used to calm the shen (mind) in Chinese medicine. It is helpful in treating anxiety, insomnia, palpitations, and forgetfulness. It is a nervine tonic and acts to nourish and strengthen the nervous system. It is helpful for treating anxiety, insomnia, palpitations, forgetfulness, nervous exhaustion, excessive stress, worry, and other heightened nervous system states.

Schisandra increases mental alertness and brain efficiency. It enhances work activity, productivity, and reflex response. It can be useful for reducing attention difficulties in children.

How to Use Schisandra

Schisandra can be enjoyed in various ways. It is popular in tea, tincture, powder, and capsule forms. It is also commonly consumed as a medicinal food. The dried berries can be eaten whole by themselves, cooked into other foods, or made into a tasty syrup.

Recommended Amounts

CAPSULES: 1 to 6 grams per day

DECOCTION: Put 1 or 2 teaspoons of dried berries into 1 to 1½ cups of water. Simmer for 5 to 10 minutes, then steep for around 25 minutes. Drink ½ cup, 3 times a day.

TINCTURE (1:2, 1:3): 2 to 5 milliliters, 2 or 3 times per day

TINCTURE (1:5): 5 milliliters, 3 times per day

Cautions and Considerations

Pregnancy Category B1: Schisandra has been traditionally contraindicated in pregnancy, except to assist in childbirth and inducing labor. However, no increase in the frequency of malformation or other harmful effects on the fetus has been found with limited use of schisandra in women.

Due to its effects on phase 1 and phase 2 liver detoxification, schisandra may accelerate the clearance of several drugs. Use with caution in combination with any pharmaceutical.

Recipes

There are many delicious ways to enjoy schisandra berries as a medicinal food. The berries can be used to make tea or cooked easily into other recipes. The powder can be added to smoothies and other drinks to increase energy and enhance detoxification.

Schisandra Berry Syrup

MAKES 4 CUPS | Prep time: 10 minutes | Cook time: 45 minutes

Schisandra berries can be made into a tasty syrup that can be poured over pancakes, added to smoothies to sweeten the taste, or eaten by the spoon. Because this syrup contains honey, it should not be given to children under the age of one.

2½ cups water   1 cup raw honey
1 cup dried schisandra berries

1. In a pot, combine the water and schisandra berries and bring to a boil. Reduce heat and simmer for 30 to 45 minutes.
2. Remove from heat and mash the berries. Strain the mixture through a cheesecloth and squeeze out all the juice, reserving it. Once cooled, add the honey and stir.
3. Store in a glass bottle or jar in the refrigerator for up to several months. Enjoy 1 to 3 (1-tablespoon) servings per day.

Detox Smoothie

**MAKES 4 (8-OUNCE) SERVINGS | Prep time: 5 minutes |
Cook time: 15 minutes**

This smoothie supports a gentle yet effective detox and is beneficial
for anyone who wants to improve their liver health and decrease their
body's total toxic burden. This recipe is especially helpful for treating
premenstrual syndrome, acne, environmental and chemical sensitivities, and liver dis-ease.

2 beets

1 cup purified water

1 cup schisandra powder

1 cup chopped organic
   dandelion greens

1 cup frozen organic berries,
   spinach, or ice (optional)

1. Fill the bottom of a steamer with 2 inches of water and bring to a
    boil. Add the beets, cover, and steam for 15 minutes. Once the beets
    are soft enough to easily insert a fork into them, set aside to cool.

2. Once cooled, peel and chop the beets. Put them into a blender with
    the purified water, schisandra powder, and dandelion greens. Add
    frozen berries, spinach, or ice (if using) as desired to modify thickness.
    Blend for about 45 seconds and serve.

3. Drink once daily for maintenance or twice daily as part of a detox
    cleanse regimen.

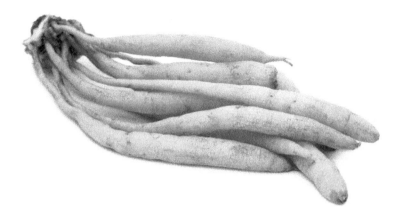

Shatavari

LATIN NAME: *Asparagus racemosus*

Shatavari is a plant native to India and the Himalayas, commonly found at high elevations of 1,200 to 1,400 meters. It is a climbing perennial, the leaves of which resemble pine needles. It grows up to 2 meters tall. It is both a sweet and bitter herb and is used in Ayurvedic medicine to cure many ailments. It is balancing to the doshas.

Be careful not to confuse this herb with its relative *Asparagus officinalis*, the asparagus we usually find on our dinner plates.

Shatavari is a powerful rasayana plant, enhancing mental and physical strength and promoting youth and longevity. It is a restorative and rejuvenating botanical that calms, cools, and nourishes the body. It is considered to be both a general nutritive tonic and a women's tonic.

Shatavari at a Glance

HELPFUL PARTS: root

ADDITIONAL NAMES: satamuli, satavari, satawar

COMMON PREPARATIONS: capsules, decoction, powder, tincture

ENERGETICS AND TASTE: bitter, cool, moist, sweet

MEDICINAL PROPERTIES: adaptogenic, antibacterial, antispasmodic, aphrodisiac, demulcent, diuretic, female reproductive tonic, galactagogue, immune tonic, lung tonic, nutritive tonic, protective to digestive tract

IDEAL FOR ADDRESSING: dry coughs, fatigue, gastrointestinal irritation, immune support, infertility, inflammation of the bladder, low breast milk production, low libido, ulcers, vaginal dryness

Benefits

WOMEN'S HEALTH: Shatavari is the most popular Ayurvedic herb for supporting women's health. It has mild hormone-balancing effects and is strengthening and nourishing to the female reproductive system. It is considered to be a uterine tonic, taken both before pregnancy to prepare the uterus for conception and during pregnancy for nourishment. Historically, this herb has been used to help prevent threatened abortions, as an aphrodisiac, and to enhance fertility.

Shatavari is commonly used to promote lactation while breast-feeding and is effective for increasing low breast milk supply. Shatavari stimulates prolactin production and release from the pituitary glands. Prolactin is the hormone that tells the body to produce breast milk.

It is a great herb for treating symptoms of menopause like vaginal dryness, low libido, dry skin, fatigue, anxiety, depression, brain fog, and insomnia.

DIGESTIVE HEALTH: Shatavari is a great herb for healing various digestive imbalances. Its demulcent, moisturizing, and cooling properties make it ideal for treating hot, inflammatory, and dry afflictions. It performs protective actions on the digestive tract and works to promote healing of irritated and inflamed tissues. It has been shown to be effective at treating gastric and duodenal ulcers. It can be taken as a powder or fresh juice to treat these afflictions. Studies performed on rats have shown that *Asparagus racemosus* is also protective for the liver and effective at regulating liver enzymes.

IMMUNE HEALTH: Just like all adaptogens, shatavari has immune-modulating and immune-enhancing effects. It has been shown to be an effective antibacterial agent against *Escherichia coli*, *Shigella dysenteriae*, *Shigella sonnei*, *Shigella flexneri*, *Vibrio cholerae*, *Salmonella* Typhi, *Pseudomonas putida*, *Bacillus subtilis*, and *Staphylococcus aureus*. It can reduce tumors in rats and also helps protect against bone marrow suppression from chemotherapy agents.

Shatavari has traditionally been used to treat various coughs and respiratory infections. It is helpful at treating dry, irritating coughs with difficult expectoration.

Shatavari is also used to treat inflammation of the bladder (interstitial cystitis) and urethra.

How to Use Shatavari

Shatavari is popularly consumed in capsule form, but it can also be enjoyed as a tincture, tea, or powder. The powder can be combined with ghee as a healthy way to incorporate this adaptogen into your diet.

Recommended Amounts

CAPSULES: 500 milligrams, 2 or 3 times per day

POWDER: up to 20 grams per day

TINCTURE (1:5): 3 to 5 milliliters, 3 times per day

DECOCTION: Add 2 teaspoons of powder to 1 cup of water. Simmer for 10 to 15 minutes, then steep for 40 minutes. Drink 1 to 2 cups per day.

Cautions and Considerations

This herb is safe to use over the long term and has no adverse effects. It is safe and beneficial to consume during pregnancy and breastfeeding.

Recipe

Shatavari Fertility Elixir

MAKES 1 CUP | Prep time: 1 minute | Cook time: 2 minutes

This elixir is a great tonic for supporting fertility and reproductive health. It can also be used to treat menopausal symptoms.

1 cup organic cow's milk, coconut milk, or almond milk

1 teaspoon shatavari powder

1 teaspoon maca powder

1 teaspoon grass-fed ghee

¼ teaspoon ground ginger

¼ teaspoon ground cinnamon

¼ teaspoon ground cardamom

Dash freshly ground black pepper

Honey (optional)

1. In a small pot, simmer the milk on low heat for about 2 minutes, stirring constantly, until it reaches 140 to 160°F. If you prefer more of a latte-style froth, you can whisk the milk while warming.
2. Mix in the shatavari, maca, ghee, ginger, cinnamon, cardamom, and pepper. Add honey (if using) to increase sweetness and add flavor.
3. Drink 1 to 2 cups per day.

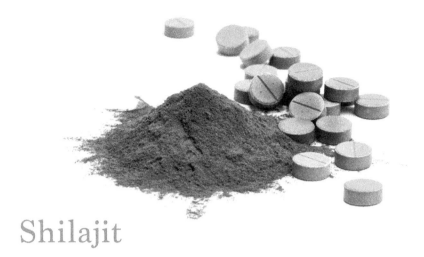

Shilajit

LATIN NAME: *Asphaltum punjabianum*

Shilajit is a natural substance that is found in the Himalayas, especially in the areas between Nepal and India. It can also be found in Russia, Tibet, and Afghanistan. It is a brownish-black exudate that seeps out between the mountain rocks in hot weather. It is believed that shilajit is formed from the decomposition of plant material over centuries. Shilajit is composed of humic and fulvic acids, which provide mineral-rich substances to soil and optimal growing environments for plants.

Shilajit is a traditional Ayurvedic rasayana, used for centuries as a rejuvenator and antiaging medicine. According to the *Charaka Samhitā*, the ancient Ayurveda medical textbook, shilajit can cure any curable disease. Shilajit is also often referred to as mumie, which in Sanskrit translates to "destroyer of weakness." In Russia, it is called mumiyo, or "mountain rock juice."

Shilajit contains more than 84 minerals, providing optimal nutrition for the body. In Nepal and Northern India, it has traditionally been given to children for breakfast to encourage healthy development and growth. It is believed to have been used by ancient Sherpa men to promote strength and longevity.

Shilajit has significant adaptogenic activity against a variety of biochemical, physiological, and psychological stressors. Research studies have shown that it exhibits antioxidant, anti-inflammatory, immune-modulating, adaptogenic, hypolipidemic, and hypoglycemic actions. It has traditionally been used in the treatment of immunological, neurological, metabolic, and urinary-tract imbalances.

Shilajit at a Glance

HELPFUL PARTS: pitch

ADDITIONAL NAMES: momia, mimijo, mumie, mumiyo, shilajeet, shilajitu

COMMON PREPARATIONS: capsules, paste, powder

ENERGETICS AND TASTE: bitter, salty, slightly pungent, warm

MEDICINAL PROPERTIES: adaptogenic, anti-inflammatory, anti-ulcer, antioxidant, hypoglycemic, immune-modulating, allergy-inhibiting

IDEAL FOR ADDRESSING: allergies, blood sugar, BPH, cognitive health, immune health, mental and physical longevity, physical and mental performance

Benefits

COGNITIVE HEALTH: According to research published in the *Indian Journal of Pharmacology* in 1992, mice given shilajit can display increased dopamine levels, enhanced learning and memory, and reduced anxiety.

Fulvic acid, one of the main active constituents of shilajit, has been found in in vitro studies to inhibit the aggregation of tau proteins, a hallmark mechanism involved in the pathogenesis of Alzheimer's disease. The same studies also showed that fulvic acid is capable of disassembling the preformed neurofibrillary tangles that make up tau proteins. This indicates that fulvic acid has the ability to both prevent and reverse tau protein formation. This research, published in the *Journal of Alzheimer's Disease* in 2011, will likely promote new insights and further research into treatments for and prevention of Alzheimer's disease.

METABOLIC AND PHYSICAL HEALTH: Shilajit can lower elevated blood sugar and improve cholesterol levels. Studies performed in mice have shown that shilajit is more effective than metformin at reducing blood sugar levels. Shilajit has also been found to reduce total and LDL cholesterol and boost HDL (the good cholesterol) levels. In an animal study published in *Hormone Molecular Biology and Clinical Investigation* in 2020, shilajit regulated liver enzymes and improved histological changes in liver cells, suggesting that it may be helpful in treating nonalcoholic fatty liver disease. Shilajit can also have anti-ulcer effects and is effective at treating gastric and duodenal ulcers.

URINARY HEALTH: One of the traditional uses of shilajit was for the removal of excess fluid from the body. Shilajit is a diuretic and has long been used in the treatment of various urinary imbalances. A Russian study of daily shilajit supplementation over a six-month period found alleviated urinary symptoms and improved objective measurements in males with benign prostatic hyperplasia (BPH).

How to Use Shilajit

Shilajit is usually enjoyed in capsule, powder, or edible paste or resin form. When consumed in edible form, it is recommended to combine shilajit with warm milk or ghee to increase absorption. It is not recommended to consume shilajit with citrus juices, as this may increase the bioavailability of aluminum in the shilajit.

Recommended Amounts

CAPSULES: 500 milligrams, 1 or 2 times per day

EDIBLE (PASTE OR RESIN): 100 to 300 milligrams, 1 or 2 times per day

POWDER: 250 to 500 milligrams, 1 or 2 times per day

Cautions and Considerations

Purified shilajit has no known toxicity or contraindications.

Unprocessed shilajit may contain heavy metals, toxic fungi, or other contaminants. When shilajit is properly purified, these contaminants are removed.

Recipe

Shilajit paste can be swallowed whole or dissolved in hot water or liquid. Shilajit is best enjoyed with ghee, coconut oil, or steamed milk.

Shilajit Power Smoothie

MAKES 1 (28-OUNCE) SMOOTHIE | Prep time: 5 minutes

This smoothie boosts energy, enhances detoxification, and improves physical and mental health. Flaxseed adds omega-3 benefits, fiber, and extra nutrition. The lignans in flaxseed act as phytoestrogens and are especially beneficial for women with hormonal imbalances.

1 cup water, coconut milk, almond milk, or goat milk

1 cup ice

½ cup organic blueberries

½ cup organic strawberries

½ cup organic blackberries

½ cup spinach leaves (optional)

250 milligrams shilajit powder

2 tablespoons flaxseed

1 tablespoon Ashwagandha Ghee (page 45) or coconut oil

Put the water, ice, blueberries, strawberries, blackberries, spinach (if using), shilajit powder, flaxseed, and ghee into a blender and process for 45 to 60 seconds, or until smooth. Serve cold and enjoy.

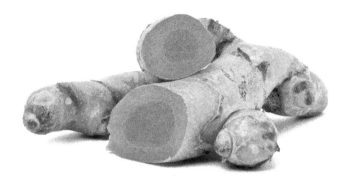

Turmeric

LATIN NAME: *Curcuma longa*

Turmeric is a tall perennial plant growing up to 1 meter high. It has large tufted leaves and pale yellow flowers. The rhizome is located internally, is oblong, and is yellow-orange in color. This plant is native to India, China, Indonesia, and other tropical areas in Southeast Asia.

Turmeric is one of the oldest cultivated spice plants in Southeast Asia. Belonging to the ginger family, it has historically been used as a spice, medicine, and topical anti-inflammatory for injuries, wounds, and inflamed joints. Its main active constituent is curcumin, which is responsible for many of the medicinal actions of the plant, including its potent anti-inflammatory effects.

Turmeric is considered to be a rasayana herb in Ayurvedic medicine, providing balance to Vata, Pitta, and Kapha constitutions. However, in excess it may aggravate Pitta and Vata states. It is used to improve circulation, cleanse the blood of toxins, purify the chakras, and support digestion, liver function, immunity, and joint health.

Turmeric was not traditionally identified as an adaptogen, but modern research has shown that it does have effects on the HPA axis and can reverse the negative effects of chronic stress. It has also been shown to increase the production of brain-derived neurotrophic factor, a protein that helps the brain repair itself, build new connections, and decrease cognitive decline. More recent studies have found that turmeric has effects on neurotransmitter balance as well and is effective at improving anxiety and depression.

Turmeric at a Glance

HELPFUL PARTS: rhizome

ADDITIONAL NAMES: acafrao, haldi, haridra, jiang huang, khamin, ukon

COMMON PREPARATIONS: capsules, decoction, edible, powder, solid extract, tincture

ENERGETICS AND TASTE: astringent, bitter, pungent, warm

MEDICINAL PROPERTIES: adaptogenic, anti-inflammatory, antioxidant, blood-thinning, carminative, cholagogue, choleretic, hepatoprotective, hypolipidemic, neuroprotectant

IDEAL FOR ADDRESSING: arthritis, autoimmune conditions, cancer prevention, cardiovascular health, inflammation, liver and gallbladder health, pain

---

Benefits

IMMUNE HEALTH: Turmeric is a natural antibiotic that strengthens digestion and improves intestinal microflora, especially in individuals with chronic weakened conditions. Studies have shown that it is also effective for treating peptic ulcer disease.

Turmeric has immune-modulating activity that down-regulates inflammatory immune reactions, making it especially helpful in the treatment of autoimmune conditions. It has also been shown to possess many cancer-preventing qualities. It is effective at inhibiting the activation of pro-carcinogenic chemicals induced by toxic agents such as cigarettes, along with several immune pathways that can trigger the proliferation of and increased blood supply to cancer cells. In vitro studies have also shown that turmeric can inhibit the proliferation of multiple myeloma cells.

PAIN AND INFLAMMATION MANAGEMENT: Turmeric is best known for its potent anti-inflammatory actions. It is commonly used in the treatment of autoimmune conditions, arthritis, joint pain, inflammatory bowel disorders, gastritis, asthma, menstrual cramps, brain inflammation, and postoperative pain.

The strongest evidence for the pain-reducing power of turmeric is its observed effects on individuals with osteoarthritis. A study published in the *Journal of Alternative and Complementary Medicine* in 2009 comparing turmeric consumption (two grams a day) with ibuprofen use over a six-week period showed that turmeric worked just as well as ibuprofen for reducing pain and inflammation in osteoarthritis of the knee. Turmeric at 2 grams per day worked just as well as NSAIDs for reducing pain.

LIVER AND GALLBLADDER HEALTH: Many of the medicinal uses of turmeric arise from its actions on the liver. It is protective to the liver thanks to its potent antioxidant and anti-inflammatory properties. It increases glutathione levels in liver cells and stimulates cellular repair. It is believed this plant may even help in the prevention of fatty liver disease, as it modulates the activity of certain mechanisms involved in its pathogenesis.

Turmeric also stimulates the formulation and release of bile from the gallbladder, which aids in the digestion and absorption of fats. This action also lowers cholesterol levels by driving the conversion of cholesterol into bile acids. Turmeric has been shown to decrease total and LDL cholesterol levels while increasing HDL cholesterol levels.

How to Use Turmeric

Turmeric is enjoyable as a tea or with warm foods or drinks. It is also commonly taken in pill and powder form, and as a tincture.

Recommended Amounts

POWDER: 1 to 4 grams, 1 or 2 times per day

STANDARDIZED EXTRACT (AT LEAST 90% CURCUMIN):
200 to 600 milligrams, 3 or 4 times per day

TINCTURE (1:1): 1 to 4 milliliters, 2 or 3 times per day

TINCTURE (1:5): 3 to 5 milliliters, 2 to 5 times per day

Cautions and Considerations

Due to its stimulating effects on the gallbladder, turmeric is contraindicated for use in cases of bile duct obstruction.

Consult with a physician before using turmeric if you are taking blood-thinning medications like warfarin or baby aspirin, as combined use may cause blood thinning and require more frequent monitoring.

As is the case for ibuprofen, turmeric should not be used the week before surgery due to its blood-thinning effects.

Recipes

Turmeric is better absorbed with fat. Black pepper, ginger, and berberine also increase absorption, so these are often paired with turmeric in recipes.

Golden Milk

MAKES 1 (12-OUNCE) SERVING | Prep time: 5 minutes | Cook time: 5 minutes

This traditional Ayurvedic recipe is great for reducing inflammation, improving cardiovascular health, supporting liver health and detoxification, lowering blood sugar, enhancing immunity, and promoting optimal health and longevity.

1½ cups full-fat coconut milk or cream

1 tablespoon coconut oil

1 to 2 teaspoons ground turmeric

½ teaspoon ground ginger

½ teaspoon ground cinnamon

Dash freshly ground black pepper

Sweetener, such as honey (optional)

In a saucepan, combine the coconut milk, coconut oil, turmeric, ginger, cinnamon, and pepper over medium heat for 4 to 5 minutes, whisking frequently. Turn off the heat, stir, and serve warm. Add more sweetener, such as honey, as desired. Enjoy 1 to 2 servings per day.

Easy and Delicious Homemade Curry

SERVES 4 | Prep time: 5 minutes | Cook time: 25 minutes

This traditional Indian recipe contains turmeric and other complementary spices that improve digestion, decrease inflammation, regulate blood sugar, and support immune and cardiovascular health. Turmeric's potent antioxidant, neuroprotective, and anticancer properties make this an ideal meal for individuals with a family or personal history of cancer, Alzheimer's disease, or cardiovascular disease. This meal is also an excellent option for individuals with chronic pain or arthritis.

- 3 cups water
- 2 cups quinoa
- 1 (13.5-ounce) can organic coconut cream
- 1 tablespoon ground cardamom
- 1 tablespoon ground coriander
- 1 tablespoon peeled finely grated fresh ginger
- 2 teaspoons ground turmeric
- 2 teaspoons ground cumin
- 1 teaspoon dry mustard
- 1 teaspoon ground cayenne pepper
- ½ teaspoon freshly ground black pepper
- 6 ounces organic firm tofu or meat
- 1 organic zucchini, sliced
- 1 cup organic broccoli florets
- 1 medium organic onion, chopped
- 1 organic red bell pepper, chopped
- ½ cup chopped fresh organic basil leaves
- 2 garlic cloves, minced
- 1 cup organic spinach
- ½ to 1 cup coconut milk (optional)

1. In a medium saucepan, bring the water to a boil. Reduce heat and add the quinoa. Cover and simmer for about 15 minutes, until the water is absorbed and the quinoa is fluffy.
2. In a large skillet or wok, combine the coconut cream, cardamom, coriander, ginger, turmeric, cumin, mustard, cayenne pepper, and black pepper. Stir well.
3. Add the tofu and simmer for 5 minutes.
4. Add the zucchini, broccoli, onion, bell pepper, basil, and garlic. Simmer and stir for 5 more minutes, until the sauce is mixed well and the vegetables are tender. Add the spinach and cook for an additional minute, until wilted. If desired, add ½ to 1 cup of additional coconut milk for a thinner curry.
5. Remove from heat and serve warm over quinoa.

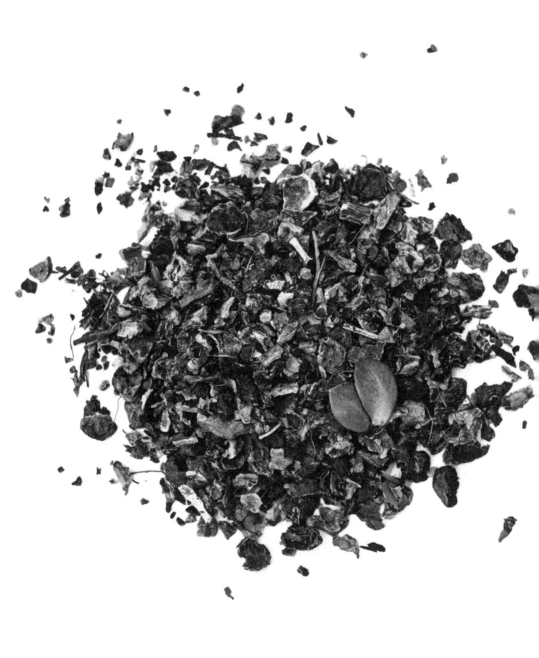

CHAPTER FIVE

Ailments and Treatments

This chapter covers several health conditions that regularly bring people to the doctor. We will discuss the common symptoms and causes of these conditions and explain how adaptogens and complementary herbs can be used in their treatment and prevention. Diet, exercise, and other healthy lifestyle recommendations will also be discussed for each condition.

Anxiety

Anxiety is the feeling we associate with our body's natural reaction to a perceived stress or threat. Occasional anxiety is something that everyone goes through and can be triggered by many different circumstances, such as tests, big events, public speaking, and major life decisions. When feelings of anxiety become excessive and persistent and interfere with everyday functioning, they are defined as anxiety disorders.

Anxiety disorders are the most common type of mental health disorder in adults. Symptoms of anxiety include excessive worry or fear, feeling overwhelmed, nervousness, and panic. Physical symptoms are also very common and include heart palpitations, shortness of breath, abdominal pain, gastrointestinal issues, trembling, and increased sweating.

The most common conventional treatment for anxiety is benzodiazepine medication. Benzodiazepines are only supposed to be prescribed for short-term use, but because of their highly addictive nature, they are often used over the long term. According to a study published in the *International Journal of Medical Sciences*, long-term use of benzodiazepines can lead to dependence, cognitive impairment, and an increased risk of developing Alzheimer's disease. Fortunately, plant adaptogens can provide an effective and much safer option for treating anxiety.

Symptoms

- Abdominal pain
- Difficulty sleeping
- Excessive worry or fear
- Fatigue
- Feeling nervous and restless
- Feeling overwhelmed or panicked
- Loose stool
- Racing heart
- Shortness of breath
- Trembling

Causes

- Adrenal fatigue
- Excessive stress
- Genetics
- Gut dysbiosis
- Hormonal imbalances
- Traumatic life events
- Underlying health issues

Treatment

Adrenal adaptogens are essential for restoring balance and function to the nervous system. Stress has been shown to inhibit neuropeptide Y, a molecule in the brain that has anxiolytic and neuroprotective effects. Adaptogens stimulate neuropeptide Y, helping relieve anxiety.

When treating anxiety, focus on calming adaptogens, as stimulating adaptogens may worsen anxiety in sensitive individuals. Some examples of calming adaptogens are ashwagandha, holy basil, schisandra, and cordyceps. These plants are helpful alone or in combination with other adaptogens and nervines. Milky oats are a great complement for anxiety treatment, as they are one of the best plants for nourishing and restoring an exhausted and depleted nervous system.

Although any of these herbs will help with anxiety, I want to highlight one specific herb. Schisandra functions as both an adaptogen and a nervine, making it an ideal candidate for the treatment of anxiety.

Schisandra dosing recommendations for anxiety:

- Tea: 1 to 2 teaspoons of berries per 1¼ cups of water, up to 3 times per day
- Tincture (1:2, 1:3): 2 to 5 milliliters, 2 or 3 times per day
- Capsules: 1 to 6 grams per day in divided doses

Regular exercise, adequate sleep, deep breathing, meditation, and mindfulness all help reduce anxiety. These lifestyle habits, along with a healthy diet, should also be included in any treatment plan to optimize your mental health.

Complementary Herbs

Magnolia

LATIN NAME: *Magnolia officinalis*

Magnolia is a deciduous tree native to China. It has been used in traditional Chinese and Japanese medicine as a warming bitter for the treatment of digestive concerns, and as a calming anxiolytic and sedative for the nervous system.

HELPFUL PARTS: bark

POPULAR PREPARATIONS: capsules, tincture

MEDICINAL PROPERTIES: anti-inflammatory, antitumor, anxiolytic, cancer protective, liver protective, neuroprotective, promotes sleep, reduces seizure activity

TIPS FOR USE: The main constituents in magnolia (honokiol and magnolo) are not readily soluble in water. Therefore, the best way to enjoy this medicine is in extract form. The therapeutic dose is 300 milligrams of magnolia extract daily, taken in divided doses. However, doses as low as 60 milligrams a day have also shown to be beneficial.

Astragalus

LATIN NAME: *Astragalus membranaceus*

Astragalus has many adaptogen-like qualities. It has been used for thousands of years in Chinese medicine. It is most well-known for its ability to enhance and modulate immune function.

HELPFUL PARTS: root

POPULAR PREPARATIONS: capsules, decoction, edible, powder, tincture

MEDICINAL PROPERTIES: antiviral, cardioprotectant, decreases fatigue, enhances tolerance to stress, immune modulator, liver protectant, strengthening tonic

TIPS FOR USE: Astragalus root is often cooked into Chinese medicinal stews. It is can be added to miso, chicken soup, bone broth, or any other nourishing soup. Cut up several slices of dried astragalus root and then simmer for 15 minutes. Other vegetables, mushrooms, or meats can then be cooked in or cooked separately and then added together.

Reishi

LATIN NAME: *Ganoderma lucidum*

Known as the "Mushroom of Immortality," Reishi is most well-known for its ability to boost and optimize immune function.

HELPFUL PARTS: mushroom, mycelial extract

POPULAR PREPARATIONS: capsules, decoction, edible, tincture

MEDICINAL PROPERTIES: anti-inflammatory, antitumor, antioxidant, antiviral, cardiac tonic, hepatoprotective, immune modulating, nervine, possible mild adaptogen

TIPS FOR USE: Add 1 cup of reishi mushrooms to a stir-fry with organic bell peppers, organic onions, organic broccoli, organic carrots, and garlic. Sauté the vegetables and mushrooms together. Once cooled, add liquid aminos or coconut aminos and ginger to taste.

Gotu Kola

LATIN NAME: *Centella asiatica*

Gotu kola is named after the Ayurvedic god Brahman for its vitality and well-being. In Ayurvedic medicine it is considered to be a brain tonic, and is tridoshic for all body types. It is called one of the "miracle elixirs of life" due to a legend of a Chinese herbalist who was said to live for over 200 years as a result of using this herb.

HELPFUL PARTS: whole plant/leaf

POPULAR PREPARATIONS: capsules, edible, fluid extract, infusion, powder extract, tincture

MEDICINAL PROPERTIES: antifibrotic, anxiolytic, circulatory tonic, nervine, nootropic, wound healing (topically)

TIPS FOR USE: Gotu kola leaves can be eaten fresh. Throw a cup of fresh gota kola leaves in with an organic spinach salad with walnuts, quinoa, and blueberries for a protein-packed and brain-boosting salad.

Depression

Depression is a mental health disorder that causes persistent feelings of low mood and sadness. Other common symptoms of depression include fatigue, indifference and lack of motivation, hopelessness, change in appetite or weight, insomnia or hypersomnia, and loss of interest or pleasure in activities once enjoyed. These symptoms interfere with normal everyday functioning and quality of life. Serious signs of depression include suicidal thoughts or ideation; when such symptoms arise, proper medical attention is necessary.

Symptoms

- Brain fog or slowed thinking
- Change in appetite
- Decreased feelings of self-worth
- Difficulty concentrating or making decisions
- Fatigue
- Fluctuations in weight
- Indifference
- Irritability
- Lack of motivation
- Loss of interest and joy
- Sadness, low mood
- Thoughts of death
- Trouble sleeping or sleeping too much

Causes

- Chronic stress
- Genetics
- Hormonal imbalances
- Inflammation
- Lack of sleep
- Neurotransmitter imbalances
- Unhealthy life situation (relationship, work)
- Unhealthy lifestyle factors (diet, lack of exercise)

Treatment

Chronic stress can be a common cause of or contributing factor to feelings of depression. Adaptogens help modulate the effects of chronic stress and have direct effects on the nervous system. These plants promote healthy mood and cognitive function. Some adaptogens are more stimulating in nature and have direct antidepressant effects on the brain.

Rhodiola is one of these stimulating adaptogens. It boosts mood by supporting the neurotransmitters dopamine, norepinephrine, and serotonin. Many clinical trials have proven its efficacy at improving mild to moderate depression. Rhaponticum is another stimulating adaptogen that is helpful for treating depression. It has been shown to be especially helpful in improving depression in recovering alcoholics. Ashwagandha, holy basil, and schisandra are considered calming adaptogens, but they also have antidepressant effects. Lemon balm is a helpful complementary herb for treating depression, as it is said to "bring joy to the heart."

Taking 340 to 680 milligrams a day of rhodiola for at least six weeks has been shown to be effective for treating mild to moderate depression. Severe depression should be evaluated and treated by a physician to ensure the most appropriate and efficacious care.

Exercise is also a great natural antidepressant. Physical activity boosts the brain's dopamine, serotonin, and norepinephrine levels, resulting in an immediate sense of euphoria and mood elevation. Aerobic exercises such as running have proven to be the most effective for alleviating depression, but any form of physical activity done on a consistent basis will provide mood-boosting benefits.

Irritability

Irritability is a feeling of agitation and being unsettled. When you are feeling irritable, you can become frustrated and annoyed more easily. Irritability can also make you more sensitive to external stimuli, as it lowers your threshold for stress. Irritability is a common symptom of chronic stress, insomnia, hormonal imbalances, blood sugar fluctuations, anxiety, and depression.

Symptoms

- Difficulty concentrating
- Emotional sensitivity
- Feeling annoyed, frustrated, or angry over trivial things
- Feelings of unease or agitation

Causes

- Adrenal fatigue
- Anxiety
- Blood sugar imbalances
- Depression
- Hormonal imbalances
- Lack of sleep
- Stress

Treatment

Irritability is a common manifestation of both acute and chronic stress. It also commonly accompanies states of anxiety and depression. A combination of adaptogens and nervines is most beneficial in treating irritability. Holy basil is a wonderful option, as it is both calming and uplifting. This adaptogenic plant enhances spiritual and emotional health, bringing calm and clarity to the mind and spirit.

Milky oats are a wonderful complementary plant for helping with irritability. They act as a nourishing nervine tonic to the mind and nervous system. Vervain is another great tonifying herb for the nervous system and is especially helpful to individuals who have a tendency to overwork and be overly self-critical.

Holy basil is best consumed as a tea to maximize its emotional and spiritual benefits. Milky oats and vervain are most therapeutic for soothing the nervous system in tincture form.

Dosing recommendations for irritability:

- Holy basil tea: 2 to 3 cups per day
- Milky oat tincture (1:2, 1:3): 2 milliliters, 3 times per day
- Vervain tincture (1:3): 1 to 3 milliliters, 3 times per day

Diaphragmatic breathing is beneficial for reducing stress and promoting emotional calm and wellness. Exercise is also an effective stress buster and mood lifter. Eating protein regularly throughout the day helps balance blood sugar levels as well, relieving irritability caused by hypoglycemia.

Low Libido

Low libido is a decreased interest in sexual activity. It is often a symptom of an underlying condition. To effectively treat reduced sexual desire, it is important to first determine the root causes of your problem. Chronic stress and hormonal imbalances are the most common physical causes of reduced libido. Psychological causes include lack of intimacy or connection, sexual dysfunction, pain with intercourse, depression, lack of confidence, and concerns with body image.

Some medications, such as antidepressants, antipsychotics, hypertension medications, and even over-the counter antihistamines, can cause decreased libido or sexual dysfunction.

Symptoms

- Reduced sexual desire

Causes

- Chronic illness
- Depression
- Fatigue
- Hormonal imbalances
- Lack of confidence
- Medication side effects
- Sexual dysfunction or pain
- Stress

Treatment

Adaptogens help restore normal reproductive function and hormonal balance. All adaptogens improve sexual drive, especially if chronic stress is the main underlying cause, but maca, Asian ginseng, and ashwagandha are especially useful for treating low libido. These herbs can be taken by both men and women; however, maca tends to be more commonly used by women, whereas Asian ginseng is the more common choice for men. Ashwagandha has a long tradition of use for improving sexual drive in both men and women.

For men, if sexual dysfunction is the cause of reduced sexual desire, Asian ginseng, American ginseng, and ashwagandha are the most effective options. For hormonal imbalances in women, rhodiola, shatavari, and maca are the most useful treatments. Schisandra has been shown to increase circulation to the genitals and enhance clitoral stimulation in women, which can be beneficial if lack of pleasure is a contributing factor. Depending on the causes of low sexual desire, these herbs can be used alone or in combination. We will spotlight maca and Asian ginseng for these concerns. Maca supplementation is best in powder or capsule form. Ginseng will be the strongest acting in tincture form.

Dosing recommendations for low libido:

- Maca powder: 3 to 5 grams per day
- Maca capsules: 1 to 2 grams per day in divided doses
- Asian ginseng tincture (1:2): 3 milliliters, 2 or 3 times per day

A healthy diet and lifestyle can also help optimize sexual desire and function. Addressing sleep imbalances, managing stress and anxiety, and improving relationship quality are effective strategies for promoting healthy libido.

Insomnia

Insomnia is defined as difficulty falling or staying asleep. Sleeping disturbances are very common, and according to the CDC, one out of every three adults does not get enough sleep to protect their health. Insomnia causes daytime fatigue and drowsiness, brain fog, and decreased mental dexterity. Long-term sleep insufficiency causes excessive inflammation in the body and can increase the risk of chronic dis-ease.

Sleep is when our brain and body reset and heal. Getting good quality and sufficient sleep is one of the most important things you can do for your health overall.

Symptoms

- Brain fog, difficulty concentrating, poor memory
- Daytime fatigue and drowsiness
- Difficulty falling asleep
- Frequent waking
- Not feeling refreshed after sleep
- Waking too early

Causes

- Alcohol
- Anxiety
- Depression
- Excessive caffeine or stimulant intake
- Hormonal imbalances
- Medication side effects
- Pain
- Stress
- Trauma or post-traumatic stress disorder

Treatment

Chronic stress is often the number-one contributing factor to sleep issues. Although all adaptogens help improve sleep through their cortisol-reducing effects and actions on the HPA axis, calming adaptogens such as schisandra, holy basil, and ashwagandha are most useful for treating insomnia and deficient sleep. Eleuthero and cordyceps are also wonderful for helping reset circadian rhythms and lower nighttime cortisol levels. There are many nervine herbs that serve as wonderful complements to adaptogens for treating insomnia. Skullcap, blue vervain, magnolia, and lemon balm are all effective at improving sleep quality and duration.

Ashwagandha and magnolia bark should be spotlighted as the herbal sleep all-star plants. Ashwagandha acts to promote both a healthy cortisol response and healthy sleep patterns. Magnolia bark decreases the time it takes to fall asleep and increases both REM and non-REM sleep stages. These herbs can be used alone but work better in combination.

Dosing recommendations for insomnia:

- Ashwagandha extract: 500 milligrams taken at night at least 30 to 60 minutes before bedtime
- Magnolia bark: 300 milligrams taken at night at least 30 to 60 minutes before bedtime

Sleep hygiene also plays an essential role in regulating healthy circadian rhythms and promoting healthy sleep patterns. Sleep hygiene includes maintaining regular sleep and wake times, reserving the bedroom for sleep and intimacy, and turning the bedroom into a sound-sleep space with darkness, cool temperatures, and reduced noise. Keeping a regular nighttime routine, shutting down all electronics at least an hour before bedtime, and avoiding stimulants and alcohol can also promote healthy sleep.

Fatigue

Fatigue is characterized by lingering feelings of mental or physical tiredness. Most people have felt fatigued at some point in their lives and are pretty familiar with the feeling. What some people may not realize, though, is that there are different types of fatigue: physical, mental, and emotional fatigue.

Low energy, reduced stamina, sleepiness, weakness, and feelings of exhaustion are common manifestations of physical fatigue. Common causes of physical fatigue include stress, poor sleep, anemia, and low thyroid function.

Mental fatigue leads to difficulties with focus and attention, reduced mental stamina, and decreased work productivity. It can be caused by overwork and is a common condition in students.

Emotional fatigue is the feeling of being emotionally worn out. This can be caused by grief, being a parent or caregiver, living with a chronic dis-ease, or many other reasons.

These forms of fatigue can be caused by chronic stress. The good news is that adaptogens can help with all of these concerns.

Symptoms

- Chronic physical and mental tiredness
- Exhaustion after mental or physical exertion
- Low energy and stamina
- Not feeling refreshed after sleep

Causes

- Anemia
- Anxiety
- Cancer or chemotherapy
- Chronic infection
- Depression
- Environmental toxins
- Food allergies
- Hypothyroidism
- Insomnia
- Medication side effects
- Stress
- Underlying health conditions

Treatment

One of the first benefits people notice when they start taking adaptogens is an improvement in their energy. Adaptogens produce a sustainable energy that increases stamina and resilience in the body. This is different than the stimulating type of "energy" that caffeine produces. Although these stimulants can reduce fatigue in the short term, they can worsen fatigue in the long run. Adaptogens can provide both immediate and long-term improvements of fatigue.

Every adaptogen discussed in this book reduces physical and mental fatigue and improves energy and stamina. To determine the best herbal treatment protocol for you, it helps to first determine the main cause of your fatigue. If insomnia is the biggest culprit, then nervines like ashwagandha are the best options. If your fatigue is caused by a chronic infection like the Epstein-Barr virus, then cordyceps and licorice are more useful. To treat cancer- or chemotherapy-induced fatigue, guduchi and astragalus are most effective.

Eleuthero is a great herb for improving general mental and physical energy. It is suitable for most individuals. To boost energy most effectively, eleuthero should be taken in tincture form.

Eleuthero dosing recommendations for fatigue:

- Tincture (1:2): 2 to 3 milliliters, 2 or 3 times per day

To further reduce fatigue, it's important to incorporate healthy lifestyle practices. A healthy diet, regular exercise, adequate sleep, and stress-reduction techniques will enhance your energy and vitality.

Poor Concentration

Poor concentration is an inability to focus your thoughts. Individuals dealing with issues of poor concentration may find it difficult to complete tasks, think clearly, or make decisions. They may also be easily distracted and have difficulty remembering things. Many factors can contribute to concentration difficulties, including stress, insufficient sleep, hormonal imbalances, food intolerances, medication side effects, mood disorders, and neurological issues.

Symptoms

- Difficulty thinking clearly
- Frequent distraction
- Inability to complete tasks or make decisions
- Lack of focus
- Problems with memory

Causes

- Attention deficit disorders
- Chronic stress
- Depression
- Environmental toxins
- Excessive technology use
- Food intolerances
- Head injuries
- Hormonal imbalances
- Insomnia
- Low blood sugar
- Medication side effects
- Recreational drug use

Treatment

All adaptogens increase mental clarity, focus, and stamina. They have neuroprotective effects and act to enhance brain function, which makes them excellent herbal choices for helping with poor concentration, brain fog, memory issues, and mental fatigue. Rhodiola has been found to increase mental stamina and improve test scores when consumed by students. Researchers are gaining interest in shilajit as a possible preventive treatment for Alzheimer's disease due to its high fulvic acid content and ability to inhibit tau protein aggregation. Holy basil is well-known for promoting spiritual and mental enlightenment. Gotu kola would be a wonderful complementary plant to add to your herbal treatment regimen as this herb increases blood flow to the brain and enhances cognition and memory.

These plants can be used alone or in combination with other adaptogens to increase concentration.

Dosing recommendations for poor concentration:

- Gotu kola tea: 1 tablespoon of leaves per 1 cup of water, 2 to 3 times per day
- Gotu kola Tincture (1:3): 3 to 5 milliliters, 3 times per day
- Shilajit capsules: 500 milligrams, 1 or 2 times per day

Exercise is a very effective way to improve focus and attention. It has been shown to stimulate the growth of new nerve cells and increase the production of neurotransmitters involved in focus and attention. A study published in the *Journal of Attention* in 2012 found that moderate to vigorous exercise 45 minutes a day three times a week improved attention and cognitive function in children with ADHD. These results, along with the results of many other studies, have shown that exercise has similar effects on the brain to ADHD medication.

Insulin Resistance

Insulin resistance arises when the body is unable to properly respond to the amount of insulin that it is producing. Insulin is produced by the pancreas to regulate the amount of sugar in the blood. When the body's blood sugar levels are consistently high, insulin resistance can occur, and if not corrected, it can lead to type 2 diabetes.

Symptoms of insulin resistance include fatigue, increased thirst or urination, blurry vision, poor wound healing, weight gain, and numbness or tingling. Insulin resistance is easily diagnosed through a blood test. Early diagnosis improves treatment outcomes and reduces the need for prescription medication.

Symptoms

- Extreme thirst or hunger
- Fatigue
- Frequent infections
- Increased or frequent urination
- Numbness or tingling in hands or feet
- Poor wound healing
- Weight gain, especially in mid-abdominal area

Causes

- Chronic conditions like polycystic ovarian disorder
- Chronic stress
- Diet high in refined carbohydrates, high-glycemic foods, and sugar
- Genetics
- Lack of sleep
- Obesity, especially increased abdominal fat
- Physical inactivity

Treatment

Chronic stress leads to increased cortisol output, which increases blood sugar levels. Persistently elevated blood sugar levels can lead to insulin resistance.

Adaptogens can help prevent this cortisol-induced blood sugar dysregulation as well as reverse stress-induced insulin resistance. All adaptogens are useful for regulating blood sugar, but of special note are American ginseng, Asian ginseng, holy basil, and shilajit. In mouse studies, shilajit was found to be more effective at lowering blood sugar levels than metformin and glibenclamide, two medications commonly used for treating type 2 diabetes. Shilajit was also shown to enhance hypoglycemic medications, and when used in combination with such medications, the greatest reductions in blood sugar were achieved.

Studies have shown that dosages of 100 milligrams/kilogram of shilajit taken once a day for four weeks are most effective at reducing blood sugar levels. It is important to note, though, that adaptogens cannot be used alone to treat type 1 diabetes, as insulin medication is indispensable for treatment of this condition.

Reducing or eliminating refined carbohydrates, high-glycemic foods, and sugar from the diet is strongly recommended for individuals working to lower and maintain blood sugar levels. Regular exercise and stress-reduction techniques are also recommended to regulate cortisol and promote a healthy stress response.

Obesity

Obesity is a condition in which excess body fat presents a risk to an individual's health. An individual with a body mass index over 30 is considered to be obese. Body mass index can be roughly calculated by dividing a person's weight in kilograms by the square of their height in meters. Obesity can increase the risk of many chronic health conditions, such as heart disease and diabetes.

Symptoms

- Fatigue
- Increased body fat

Causes

- Chronic health conditions like diabetes
- Chronic stress
- Diet choices
- Genetics
- Hormonal imbalances
- Inactivity or lack of exercise
- Poor sleep

Treatment

Adaptogens help promote a healthy stress response, working physically to restore balance in the body and psychologically to control stress-induced binge eating or alcohol consumption. Adaptogens also support weight management by helping regulate blood sugar, insulin, and cortisol levels; improve sleep; and optimize metabolism. Every adaptogen discussed in this book supports healthy weight management.

Although adaptogens may not be magic weight-loss pills, they do help reverse and prevent many common physiological imbalances that lead to weight gain. There are many complementary herbs that can also be helpful for addressing these imbalances. These plants should be used as a supplement to your health plan along with diet and exercise.

Avoiding foods that are highly processed, high in sugar, high in trans fats, inflammatory, or devoid of nutrients is essential to managing healthy weight. A whole-foods diet focused on organic vegetables and fruits and healthy fats and proteins is recommended. There are several different therapeutic diets marketed for helping with weight loss. The key is finding the diet that works for you. Just like everything else, there is no one-size-fits-all diet. However, if you avoid fast foods, junk foods, and excessive alcohol consumption, you're on the right track.

Both aerobic and anaerobic exercises support healthy weight management. Aerobic exercises such as running, biking, swimming, and walking will burn calories, whereas anaerobic exercises such as weight training increase lean muscle mass, improve metabolism, and increase fat burning. Combining aerobic and anaerobic exercise has been found to be the most effective way to achieve weight loss. Studies have also shown that interval training, which involves short periods of intense exercise, maximizes these weight-loss benefits.

Hypertension (High Blood Pressure)

Hypertension is defined as a blood pressure at or above 130 systolic and 80 diastolic. High blood pressure involves long-term force of the blood against artery walls. This can lead to heart disease, stroke, or other health conditions if left untreated.

Hypertension is usually asymptomatic, and it is often only detected through blood pressure readings. Possible symptoms of hypertension include headaches, shortness of breath, and nosebleeds. These symptoms are typically only seen in chronically uncontrolled hypertensive states and are nonspecific to the condition.

Symptoms

- Headaches
- Nosebleeds
- Shortness of breath

Causes

- Chronic health conditions like diabetes, heart disease, and sleep apnea
- Chronic kidney dis-ease
- Chronic stress
- Cigarette smoking
- Diet high in salt and low in potassium
- Genetics
- High alcohol consumption
- Obesity
- Pregnancy
- Sedentary lifestyle

Treatment

All adaptogens can help improve blood pressure through their stress-modulating and normalizing effects on the body. Holy basil and cordyceps have been shown to be especially effective at lowering blood pressure. Holy basil has a hypotensive vasodilatory effect, is cardioprotective, and has been shown to inhibit platelet aggregation and clotting time. Cordyceps is also believed to have vasodilatory effects and has been shown to be effective at treating mild hypertension. It can also normalize heart arrhythmias, decrease blood viscosity, and improve cardiac function. Cordyceps is especially recommended for treating blood pressure issues caused by kidney dysfunction, as it is effective for strengthening and restoring healthy kidney function. Gotu kola is another great herb for enhancing circulation and reducing blood pressure.

Cordyceps dosing recommendations for hypertension:

- Tincture (1:4, 1:5): 1 to 2 milliliters, 3 times per day
- Edible (cooked whole mushroom): 1 cup, 2 times per day

Depending on the severity of hypertension, these herbs can be used alone or in conjunction with blood pressure medications. As hypertension by itself is asymptomatic, it is important to visit the doctor regularly to have this concern properly evaluated. If you have increased risk factors for hypertension, you may want to invest in an at-home blood pressure machine to regularly check your readings.

Exercise is an important lifestyle factor for helping lower and maintain blood pressure levels. To achieve these positive cardiovascular effects, 30 minutes of aerobic exercise on most days of the week is recommended. This can include walking, biking, running, climbing stairs, playing sports, dancing, or swimming.

Eating a healthy diet low in sodium, reducing alcohol consumption, and quitting smoking are also effective lifestyle changes for naturally reducing blood pressure. Yoga, meditation, and breathing exercises can reduce stress and improve cardiovascular function as well.

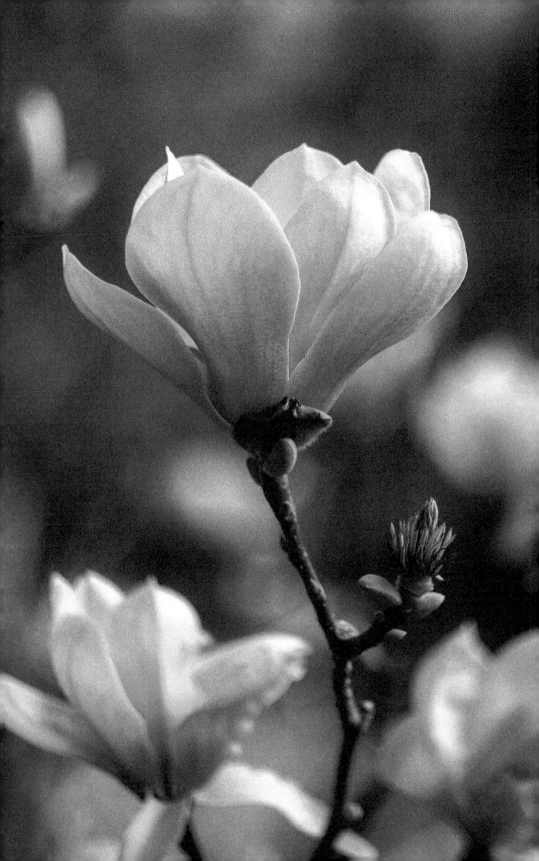

CHAPTER SIX

Complementary Practices: Help the Plants Help You

This last chapter offers lifestyle recommendations to complement your adaptogen-based health program. The techniques described here have been well researched for their benefits of reducing stress, elevating mood, improving mental clarity, and enhancing overall health. These lifestyle modifications enhance the effects of adaptogens, helping you achieve and maintain optimal health, vitality, and longevity.

Self-Inquiry

Although it's nice to have tools to modulate our stress response, it is just as important to identify and remove major stressors in our lives, as these can be obstacles in the path to healing.

Major stresses in our lives can easily lead to feelings of being overwhelmed, anxiety, and exhaustion. Modern life has made stress the new normal, and we often don't take the time to identify what our stressors are and how they are affecting us. Unfortunately, this stress doesn't become apparent to many people until they crash with adrenal exhaustion. Taking the time to reflect and identify your stressors now will help you implement healthy lifestyle modifications to prevent future adrenal burnout and stress-induced chronic dis-ease.

Ideally, removal of these major obstacles is the best solution for promoting health and wellness. However, this is not always possible. Fortunately, there are many ways you can modulate the effects of stressors. Exercise, breathing techniques, yoga, meditation, and journaling are very effective tools for reducing stress and improving physical and emotional health.

Mindset plays a critical role in regulating the effects of stress. Many studies have shown that a positive mindset improves health, wellness, and longevity. One easy way to shift your mindset to focus more on the positives in your life is by practicing gratitude.

Studies have shown that people who express gratitude on a regular basis experience more positive emotions, have improved self-esteem, have better-quality sleep, and overall enjoy better emotional and physical health. Practicing gratitude helps negate toxic emotions, improves self-worth, and can help you attain personal goals.

Experiencing gratitude also increases your resilience to stress and trauma, helping you bounce back quicker and more effectively from stressful events. An attitude of thankfulness can both decrease susceptibility to and heal the negative psychological effects of a traumatic event.

Just like everything else, expressing gratitude takes practice. A good place to start is spending a few minutes every day reflecting on one thing you are grateful for. It doesn't have to be something big or grand. In fact, by routinely expressing gratitude for the little things in life, you'll realize just how great your life actually is. Some examples of things we might take for granted include a sunny day, a good night's sleep, a good song on the radio, or anything that makes us smile. If you can start feeling grateful for these little everyday things, you'll be able to live a happier and more resilient life.

Breath Work

Controlling your breath is one of the quickest and most powerful ways to negate the stress response and promote relaxation. Deep, diaphragmatic breathing stimulates the vagus nerve, which plays a vital role in regulating the autonomic nervous system. Remember that sympathetic "fight or flight" response that is triggered when we first perceive a stressor? The vagus nerve is the part of the parasympathetic nervous system that acts to shut down that sympathetic stress response. Modification of this autonomic stress response stops the release of cortisol and other stress hormones, preventing a state of chronic stress.

Diaphragmatic breathing involves learning how to slow and deepen the breath. Most people tend to breathe from the chest and as a result have shallower and quicker breathing. Anxiety and acute stressors can cause the sympathetic nervous system to exaggerate this superficial breathing pattern and lead to feelings of hyperventilation and shortness of breath. By taking deeper and slower breaths, you activate the parasympathetic nervous system, which then sends messages to the brain and body to calm down and relax.

The way you breathe affects your whole body, and learning to control and slow down your breath is one of the best things you can do to improve your health. Diaphragmatic breathing reduces heart rate and blood pressure and improves cardiovascular function. Clinically, this breathing technique is a form of biofeedback that improves heart rate variability. Heart rate variability is variation in the time between heartbeats. Higher heart rate variability is associated with increased resilience to stress, healthy cardiovascular function, and optimal health.

There are many different therapeutic breathing techniques, but the easiest one to start out with is belly breathing. This is another name for diaphragmatic breathing, and it involves taking deep belly breaths. If you tend to run on the anxious side, belly breathing exercises may be difficult for you; I recommend starting off slow and gradual. Try taking one minute at the end of your day to sit, relax, and focus on slowing your breathing, taking deep inhalations into long exhalations and breathing from your belly instead of your chest. Lying down in bed and putting one hand on your chest and one hand on your abdomen may help you train your brain where to breathe from. Another trick is to place a light book on your abdomen and try to push it upward with each inhalation. Once you learn the proper techniques, increase the frequency with which you practice these breaths. If you have digestive issues, a few minutes of deep, slow breathing will improve your digestion and absorption of nutrients. The more you practice these breathing techniques, the more natural and autonomic they will become.

Yoga

Yoga is an excellent complementary exercise to add to your plant-based healing program as it provides amazing benefits to the body, mind, and spirit. Yoga practices incorporate movement, therapeutic breathing, and mindfulness techniques that promote parasympathetic function. Yoga has become a popular form of exercise for reducing stress and improving physical fitness, but its health benefits reach far beyond that.

Yoga has been practiced for thousands of years to unite the body, mind, and spirit. It is believed to help people achieve spiritual awakening and enlightenment, bringing harmony between human beings and nature. Yoga soothes tension in the body and mind, fostering spiritual and personal development.

These ancient healing practices cultivate deeper mind-body awareness and improve both psychological and physiological health. Yogic breathing exercises bring the body out of stress mode and into a state of relaxation. This helps calm the mind, improve lung and cardiovascular health, and decrease inflammation in the body. Regular yoga practice has been shown to lower cholesterol, blood pressure, and blood sugar levels. Yoga, combined with other forms of exercise, will support a heart-healthy lifestyle. Yoga is also strengthening to the muscles, bones, and joints, enhancing flexibility, posture, and balance. Yogic movements improve circulation, encourage lymphatic drainage, and boost immunity. Many athletes find that adding yoga to their rigorous training regimens improves their flexibility, coordination, and mental fitness.

Yoga practices have been shown to reduce symptoms of anxiety, depression, and overall psychological stress. These practices bring clarity to the mind and improve focus and attention. Brain-imaging scans have found that regular yoga practice actually causes structural and functional changes to the brain, increasing blood flow and plasticity. Brain plasticity refers to the brain's ability to change, adapt, and rewire itself, and this phenomenon is essential for healthy brain development and recovery from traumatic brain injury.

The practice of mindfulness during yoga will begin to translate into other areas of your life, leading to reduced feelings of stress, increased frequency of positive experiences, better sleep, and healthier diet and lifestyle choices.

Incorporating these movements, breathing techniques, and mindfulness practices into your life can be transformative. Regular practice of yoga will help you achieve and maintain your wellness goals.

Massage

Massage is a popular practice for relieving stress. It reduces our stress hormone levels and stimulates the release of endorphins, the chemicals that make us feel happy. These effects improve our overall sense of wellness and peace. Massage is beneficial to mental health and has been shown to improve depression, anxiety, and sleep quality.

Stress reduction is the number one reason people seek out massage therapy. The physical pressure delivered through massage increases vagal activity, halting the stress response and promoting deep relaxation through activation of the parasympathetic nervous system. Levels of cortisol, norepinephrine, and adrenaline decrease, and serotonin and dopamine levels increase. These effects bring instant relaxation to the body and the mind. Massage treatments also support healthy cardiovascular function and can lower heart rate and blood pressure.

Massage has been practiced for thousands of years. It was one of the earliest forms of treatment for pain reduction, and it is still commonly used for that purpose today. Massage therapy is beneficial for treating injuries and muscle aches and pains, reducing scar tissue, and improving joint mobility. Regular massage treatments have been shown to improve fibromyalgia, temporomandibular joint (TMJ) dysfunction, headaches, and other chronic pain conditions. It is a favorite complementary treatment of athletes, who rely on massage to reduce muscle soreness, speed up recovery time, and treat and prevent injuries.

Massage techniques improve circulation and promote lymphatic movement and drainage. The lymphatic system plays a major role in supporting our immune and detoxification systems. It helps the body get rid of toxins, waste, and other unwanted materials. It also transports fluids containing white blood cells to help the body fight off infections. Massage promotes healthy lymphatic movement and drainage in the body. This is why you are told to drink lots of water after receiving a massage as hydration helps flush out the toxins mobilized. Massage therapy is often used in cancer care hospitals and clinics as a complementary treatment for these immune and detoxification benefits.

Studies have shown that the effects of massage are additive and regular treatment provides more sustainable health benefits. Adding massage therapy to your adaptogen wellness program will further support your vitality and well-being.

Meditation

Meditation is a wonderful way to help reduce stress. Many people struggle with meditation because they think that meditation means they need to quiet their mind. This is a huge myth. Meditation, by definition, is a way to transform your thoughts, not quiet them. Through meditation you gain perspective on what is happening in your mind and body, or mindfulness. Mindfulness is essentially being present to the current moment, what is happening in your body and what is around you, and not being overly reactive to or overwhelmed by your environment. It helps you learn to not dwell on what happened yesterday or worry about what tomorrow brings. You don't need to have special skills to meditate or be mindful; you just need practice.

Many of the health benefits associated with yoga are attributed to its meditative practices. Meditation practices help reduce stress, boost concentration, improve mood, and enhance mental performance.

There are many ways to practice meditation and mindfulness. If you're just starting out, it can be easy to get discouraged and feel like you're not doing it right. Remember, meditation doesn't mean erasing the mind; it means being present. Start slowly and gradually build up your meditative practice. There are many smartphone applications and guided meditations online that can help you get started. Dr. Inna Khazan, Dr. Jon Kabat-Zinn, and Zen Master Thich Nhat Hanh are wonderful mentors to follow. Headspace, Calm, and Insight Timer are among the most popular smartphone meditation apps. Yoga and meditation classes are also great options. The most important thing is finding what works best for you.

Medical Terms Glossary

Amphoteric: normalizes function in a tissue or organ

Anodyne: relieves pain, especially nerve pain

Anti-anxiolytic: antianxiety

Antipyretic: fever-reducing

Carminative: relieves gastrointestinal cramping and expels gas

Chemoprotective: protects the body from the side effects of chemotherapy

Cholagogue: helps bile flow, which has a mild laxative effect.

Choleretic: stimulates production of bile

Demulcent: protects mucous membranes and soothes irritation

Diaphoretic: promotes sweating

Expectorant: brings up mucus from the airways

Galactagogue: stimulates breast milk production

Hepatoprotective: protects against liver damage

Hypolipidemic: lowers lipid levels

Immune-modulating: alters or regulates immune system function

Nervine: soothes, strengthens, and restores normal function to the nervous system

Neuroprotectant: protects the brain against cell injury/death, degeneration, stroke, and toxins

Nootropic: increases cerebral blood flow and enhances memory

Phytoestrogen: A plant component that mimics the effects of estrogen hormones in the body.

Thyroiditis: Inflammation of the thyroid gland. Includes Hashimoto's thyroiditis, subacute thyroiditis, and postpartum or silent thyroiditis.

Resources

For further information on adaptogens and other botanical medicines, the following resources are recommended.

Books:

300 Herbs: Their Indications & Contraindications (A Materia Medica & Repertory) by Matthew Alfs, MH, RH (AHG)

Adaptogens: Herbs for Strength, Stamina, and Stress Relief by David Winston, RH (AHG), and Steven Maimes

Adaptogens in Medical Herbalism: Elite Herbs and Natural Compounds for Mastering Stress, Aging, and Chronic Disease by Donald R. Yance, CN, MH, RH (AHG), SFO

Ayurvedic Herbs: The Comprehensive Resource for Ayurvedic Healing Solutions by Virender Sodhi, MD, ND

Herbal Medicine: From the Heart of the Earth by Sharol Tilgner, ND

Medical Herbalism: The Science and Practice of Herbal Medicine by David Hoffmann, FNIMH, RH (AHG)

Medicinal Mushrooms: An Exploration of Tradition, Healing, and Culture by Christopher Hobbs, PhD, LAc

Websites:

AMERICAN BOTANICAL COUNCIL: HerbalGram.org

HENRIETTE'S HERBAL HOMEPAGE: Henriettes-Herb.com

SOUTHWEST SCHOOL OF BOTANICAL MEDICINE:
SWSBM.com/HOMEPAGE/HomePage.html

For trusted sources for purchasing your adaptogenic or other botanical medicines:

BANYAN BOTANICALS: BanyanBotanicals.com

GAIA HERBS: GaiaHerbs.com

HERB PHARM: Herb-Pharm.com

MOUNTAIN ROSE HERBS: MountainRoseHerbs.com

REBEL HERBS: RebelHerbs.com

WISE WOMAN HERBALS: WiseWomanHerbals.com

Note: I have no financial affiliation with any of these organizations.

References

Afanasjeva, T. N., A. A. Krivchik, and T. P. Murtasova, ed. *New Data on Eleuthercoccus: Proceedings of the Second International Symposium on Eleutherococcus.* Moscow: Academy of Sciences of the USSR Far East Science Center, 1985.

Ahmad, Mohammad Kaleem, Abbas Ali Mahdi, Kamla Kant Shukla, Najmul Islam, Singh Rajender, Dama Madhukar, Satya Narain Shankhwar, and Sohail Ahmad. "*Withania somnifera* Improves Semen Quality by Regulating Reproductive Hormone Levels and Oxidative Stress in Seminal Plasma of Infertile Males." *Fertility and Sterility* 94, no. 3 (August 2010): 989–996.

Ai, Zhong, Ai-Fang Cheng, Yuan-Tao Yu, Long-Jiang Yu, and Wenwen Jin. "Antidepressant-Like Behavioral, Anatomical, and Biochemical Effects of Petroleum Ether Extract from Maca (*Lepidium meyenii*) in Mice Exposed to Chronic Unpredictable Mild Stress." *Journal of Medicinal Food* 17, no. 5 (May 2014): 535–542. doi: 10.1089/jmf.2013.2950.

Al-Qarawi, Ali A., H. A. Abdel-Rahman, Badreldin H. Ali, and Samy A. El-Mougy. "Liquorice (*Glycyrrhiza glabra*) and the Adrenal-Kidney-Pituitary Axis in Rats." *Food and Chemical Toxicology* 40, no. 10 (October 2002): 1525–1527.

Archana, R., and A. Namasivayam. "Antistressor Effect of *Withania somnifera*." *Journal of Ethnopharmacology* 64, no. 1 (January 1999): 91–93. doi:10.1016/s0378-8741(98)00107-x.

Armanini, D., I. Karbowiak, and J. W. Funder. "Affinity of Liquorice Derivatives for Mineralocorticoid and Glucocorticoid Receptors." *Clinical Endocrinology* 19 (November 1983): 609–612.

Asano, K., T. Takahashi, M. Miyashita, A. Matsuzaka, S. Muramatsu, M. Kuboyama, H. Kugo, and J. Imai. "Effect of *Eleutherococcus senticosus* Extract on Human Physical Working Capacity." *Planta Medica,* no. 3 (June 1986): 175–177.

Badar, V. A., V. R. Thawani, P. T. Wakode, M. P. Shrivastava, K. J. Gharpure, L. L. Hingorani, and R. M. Khiyani. "Efficacy of *Tinospora cordifolia* in Allergic Rhinitis." *Journal of Ethnopharmacology* 96, no. 3 (January 2005): 445–449.

Bhattacharya, S. K., A. Bhattacharya, K. Sairam, and S. Ghosal. "Anxiolytic-Antidepressant Activity of *Withania somnifera* Glycowithanolides: An Experimental Study." *Phytomedicine: International Journal of Phytotherapy and Phytopharmacology* 7, no. 6 (December 2000): 463–469. doi:10.1016/S0944-7113(00)80030-6.

Brekhman, I. I., and I. V. Dardymov. "New Substances of Plant Origin Which Increase Nonspecific Resistance." *Annual Review of Pharmacology* 9 (1969): 419–430. doi:10.1146/annurev.pa.09.040169.002223.

Brown, Richard P., Patricia L. Gerbarg, and Zakir Ramazanov. "*Rhodiola rosea*: A Phytomedicinal Overview." *HerbalGram*, no. 56 (Fall 2002): 40–52.

Bystritsky, Alexander, Lauren Kerwin, and Jamie D. Feusner. "A Pilot Study of *Rhodiola rosea* (Rhodax) for Generalized Anxiety Disorder (GAD)." *Journal of Alternative and Complementary Medicine (New York, NY)* 14, no. 2 (March 2008): 175–180. doi:10.1089/acm.2007.7117.

Carrasco-Gallardo, Carlos, Leonardo Guzmán, and Ricardo B. Maccioni. "Shilajit: A Natural Phytocomplex with Potential Procognitive Activity." *International Journal of Alzheimer's Disease* 2012 (February 2012): 674142. doi:10.1155/2012/674142.

Cornejo, Alberto, José M. Jiménez, Leonardo Caballero, Francisco Melo, and Ricardo B. Maccioni. "Fulvic Acid Inhibits Aggregation and Promotes Disassembly of Tau Fibrils Associated with Alzheimer's Disease." *Journal of Alzheimer's Disease* 27, no. 1 (October 2011): 143–153. doi:10.3233/JAD-2011-110623.

"*Curcuma longa* (Turmeric). Monograph." *Alternative Medicine Review* 6 (September 2001): S62–S66.

Darbinyan, V., G. Aslanyan, E. Amroyan, E. Gabrielyan, C. Malmström, and A. Panossian. "Clinical Trial of *Rhodiola rosea L.* Extract SHR-5 in the Treatment of Mild to Moderate Depression." *Nordic Journal of Psychiatry* 61, no. 5 (2007): 343–348. [Published correction appears in *Nordic Journal of Psychiatry* 61, no. 6 (2007): 503.] doi:10.1080/08039480701643290.

Davydov, Marina, and Abraham D. Krikorian. "*Eleutherococcus senticosus* (Rupr. & Maxim.) Maxim. (Araliaceae) as an Adaptogen: A Closer Look." *Journal of Ethnopharmacology* 72, no. 3 (October 2000): 345–393.

de Andrade, Enrico, Alexandre A. de Mesquita, Joaquim de Almeida Claro, Priscila M. de Andrade, Valdemar Ortiz, Mário Paranhos, and Miguel Srougi. "Study of the Efficacy of Korean Red Ginseng in the Treatment of Erectile Dysfunction." *Asian Journal of Andrology* 9, no. 2 (March 2007): 241–244.

Dhama, Kuldeep, Swati Sachan, Rekha Khandia, Ashok Munjal, Hafiz M. N. Iqbal, Shyma K. Latheef, Kumaragurubaran Karthik, Hari A. Samad, Ruchi Tiwari, and Maryam Dadar. "Medicinal and Beneficial Health Applications of *Tinospora cordifolia* (Guduchi): A Miraculous Herb Countering Various Diseases/ Disorders and Its Immunomodulatory Effects." *Recent Patents on Endocrine, Metabolic & Immune Drug Discovery* 10, no. 2 (2017): 96–111. doi:10.2174/1872214811666170301105101.

"*Eleutherococcus senticosus* (Rupr. & Maxim.) Maxim." in *The ABC Clinical Guide to Herbs*, edited by Mark Blumenthal, 97–106. Austin: American Botanical Council, 2003.

Felter, Harvey Wickes, and John Uri Lloyd. *King's American Dispensatory.* 18th ed. Cincinnati: Ohio Valley Co., 1898.

Fiore, Cristina, Michael Eisenhut, Rea Krausse, Eugenio Ragazzi, Donatella Pellati, Decio Armanini, and Jens Bielenberg. "Antiviral Effects of *Glycyrrhiza* Species." *Phytotherapy Research* 22, no. 2 (February 2008): 141–148. doi:10.1002/ptr.2295.

Fu, Ying, and Li Li Ji. "Chronic Ginseng Consumption Attenuates Age-Associated Oxidative Stress in Rats." *The Journal of Nutrition* 133, no. 11 (November 2003): 3603–3609. doi:10.1093/jn/133.11.3603.

Gerasimova, H. D. "Effect of *Rhodiola rosea* Extract on Ovarian Functional Activity." In *Proceedings of Scientific Conference on Endocrinology and Gynecology*, 46–48. Siberia: Siberian Branch of the Russian Academy of Sciences, 1970.

Ghezelbash, Baran, Nader Shahrokhi, Mohammad Khaksari, Firouz Ghaderi-Pakdel, and Gholamreza Asadikaram. "Hepatoprotective Effects of Shilajit on High Fat-Diet Induced Non-Alcoholic Fatty Liver Disease (NAFLD) in Rats." *Hormone Molecular Biology and Clinical Investigation* 41, no. 1 (February 2020). doi:10.1515/hmbci-2019-0040.

Gray, Nora E., Armando Alcazar Magana, Parnian Lak, Kirsten M. Wright, Joseph Quinn, Jan F. Stevens, Claudia S. Maier, and Amala Soumyanath. "*Centella asiatica*: Phytochemistry and Mechanisms of Neuroprotection and Cognitive Enhancement." *Phytochemistry Reviews: Proceedings of the Phytochemical Society of Europe* 17, no. 1 (February 2018): 161–194. doi:10.1007/s11101-017-9528-y.

Guo, Shan-Shan, Xiao-Fang Gao, Yan-Rong Gu, Zhong-Xiao Wan, A-Ming Lu, Zheng-Hong Qin, and Li Luo. "Preservation of Cognitive Function by *Lepidium meyenii* (Maca) Is Associated with Improvement of Mitochondrial Activity and Upregulation of Autophagy-Related Proteins in Middle-Aged Mouse Cortex." *Evidence-Based Complementary and Alternative Medicine* 2016 (2016): 4394261. doi:10.1155/2016/4394261.

Jaiswal, Arun Kumar, and S. K. Bhattacharya. "Effects of Shilajit on Memory, Anxiety and Brain Monoamines in Rats." *Indian Journal of Pharmacology* 24 (January 1992): 12–17.

Jeyachandran, R., T. Francis Xavier, and S. P. Anand. "Antibacterial Activity of Stem Extracts of *Tinospora Cordifolia* (Willd) Hook. f & Thomson." *Ancient Science of Life* 23, no. 1 (July 2003): 40–43.

Jorgensen, B. B. "Glycyrrhetinic Acid in Dermatological Treatment." *Acta Dermato-Venereologica* 38, no. 3 (1958): 189–193.

Kim, Seung Hwan, and Kyung Shin Park. "Effects of *Panax ginseng* Extract on Lipid Metabolism in Humans." *Pharmacological Research* 48, no. 5 (November 2003): 511–513. doi:10.1016/s1043-6618(03)00189-0.

Klepser, Teresa, and Nicole Nisly. "Astragalus as an Adjunctive Therapy in Immunocompromised Patients." *Integrative Medicine Alert* 2 (November 1999): 125–128.

Kuo, Jip, Kenny Wen-Chyuan Chen, I-Shiung Cheng, Pu-Hsi Tsai, Ying-Jui Lu, and Ning-Yuean Lee. "The Effect of Eight Weeks of Supplementation with *Eleutherococcus senticosus* on Endurance Capacity and Metabolism in Human." *Chinese Journal of Physiology* 53, no. 2 (April 2010): 105–111. doi:10.4077/cjp.2010.amk018.

Kuptniratsaikul, Vilai, Sunee Thanakhumtorn, Pornsiri Chinswang-watanakul, Luksamee Wattanamongkonsil, and Visanu Thamlikitkul. "Efficacy and Safety of *Curcuma domestica* Extracts in Patients with Knee Osteoarthritis." *Journal of Alternative and Complementary Medicine (New York, NY)* 15, no. 8 (August 2009): 891–897. doi:10.1089/acm.2008.0186.

Lim, Hyun-Woo, Young-Min Kwon, Su-Min Cho, Jee-Hun Kim, Gyu-Hyung Yoon, Seung-Jung Lee, Ha-Won Kim, and Min-Won Lee. "Antitumor Activity of *Cordyceps militaris* on Human Cancer Cell Line." *Korean Journal of Pharmacognosy* 35, no. 4 (December 2004): 364–367.

Medina, José A., Turibio L. B. Netto, Mauro Muszkat, Afonso C. Medina, Denise Botter, Rogério Orbetelli, Luzia F. C. Scaramuzza, Elaine G. Sinnes, Márcio Vilela, and Mônica C. Miranda. "Exercise Impact on Sustained Attention of ADHD Children, Methylphenidate Effects." *Attention Deficit and Hyperactivity Disorders* 2, no. 1 (March 2010): 49–58. doi:10.1007/s12402-009-0018-y.

Mehta, A. K., P. Binkley, S. S. Gandhi, and M. K. Ticku. "Pharmacological Effects of *Withania somnifera* Root Extract on GABAA Receptor Complex." *Indian Journal of Medical Research* 94 (August 1991): 312–315.

Meissner, H. O., P. Mrozikiewicz, T. Bobkiewicz-Kozlowska, A. Mscisz, B. Kedzia, A. Lowicka, H. Reich-Bilinska, W. Kapczynski, and I. Barchia. "Hormone-Balancing Effect of Pre-Gelatinized Organic Maca (*Lepidium peruvianum* Chacon): (I) Biochemical and Pharmacodynamic Study on Maca Using Clinical Laboratory Model on Ovariectomized Rats." *International Journal of Biomedical Science* 2, no. 3 (September 2006): 260–272.

Mills, Simon, and Kerry Bone. *Principles and Practice of Phytotherapy: Modern Herbal Medicine*. London: Churchill Livingstone, 1999.

Mills, Simon, and Kerry Bone. *The Essential Guide to Herbal Safety*. London: Churchill Livingstone, 2004.

Mondal, Shankar, Saurabh Varma, Vishwa Deepak Bamola, Satya Narayan Naik, Bijay Ranjan Mirdha, Madan Mohan Padhi, Nalin Mehta, and Sushil Chandra Mahapatra. "Double-Blinded Randomized Controlled Trial for Immunomodulatory Effects of Tulsi (*Ocimum sanctum* Linn.) Leaf Extract on Healthy Volunteers." *Journal of Ethnopharmacology* 136, no. 3 (July 2011): 452–456. doi:10.1016/j.jep.2011.05.012.

Nair, Rajesh, Senthy Sellaturay, and Seshadri Sriprasad. "The History of Ginseng in the Management of Erectile Dysfunction in Ancient China (3500–2600 BCE)." *Indian Journal of Urology: Journal of the Urological Society of India* 28, no. 1 (January 2012): 15–20. doi:10.4103/0970-1591.94946.

Panda, Ashok Kumar, and Kailash Chandra Swain. "Traditional Uses and Medicinal Potential of *Cordyceps sinensis* of Sikkim." *Journal of Ayurveda and Integrative Medicine* 2, no. 1 (January 2011): 9–13. doi:10.4103/0975-9476.78183.

Panossian, Alexander, and Georg Wikman. "Effects of Adaptogens on the Central Nervous System and the Molecular Mechanisms Associated with Their Stress-Protective Activity." *Pharmaceuticals (Basel, Switzerland)* 3, no. 1 (January 2010): 188–224. doi:10.3390/ph3010188.

Panossian, Alexander, and Georg Wikman. "Evidence-Based Efficacy of Adaptogens in Fatigue, and Molecular Mechanisms Related to Their Stress-Protective Activity." *Current Clinical Pharmacology* 4, no. 3 (September 2009): 198–219. doi:10.2174/157488409789375311.

Panossian, Alexander, and Hildebert Wagner. "Adaptogens: A Review of Their History, Biological Activity, and Clinical Benefits." *HerbalGram* 90 (Summer 2011): 52–63.

Panossian, Alexander, Georg Wikman, Punit Kaur, and Alexzander Asea. "Adaptogens Exert a Stress-Protective Effect by Modulation of Expression of Molecular Chaperones." *Phytomedicine: International Journal of Phytotherapy and Phytopharmacology* 16, no. 6–7 (June 2009): 617–622. doi:10.1016/j.phymed.2008.12.003.

Panossian, Alexander, Georg Wikman, Punit Kaur, and Alexzander Asea. "Adaptogens Stimulate Neuropeptide Y and Hsp72 Expression and Release in Neuroglia Cells." *Frontiers in Neuroscience* 6 (February 2012): 6. doi: 10.3389/fnins.2012.00006.

Park, Hyun Jun, Sangmin Choe, and Nam Cheol Park. "Effects of Korean Red Ginseng on Semen Parameters in Male Infertility Patients: A Randomized, Placebo-Controlled, Double-Blind Clinical Study." *Chinese Journal of Integrative Medicine* 22, no. 7 (July 2016): 490–495. doi:10.1007/s11655-015-2139-9.

Physicians' Desk Reference (PDR) for Herbal Medicines. Montvale, NJ: Medical Economics Company, 2001.

Pompei, R., O. Flore, M. A. Marccialis, A. Pani, and B. Loddo. "Glycyrrhizic Acid Inhibits Virus Growth and Inactivates Virus Particles." *Nature* 281, no. 5733 (October 1979): 689–690. doi:10.1038/281689a0.

Qian, Xi-Jing, Xiao-Lian Zhang, Ping Zhao, Yong-Sheng Jin, Hai-Sheng Chen, Qing-Qiang Xu, Hao Ren, et al. "A Schisandra-Derived Compound Schizandronic Acid Inhibits Entry of Pan-HCV Genotypes into Human Hepatocytes." *Scientific Reports* 6 (June 2016): 27268. doi:10.1038/srep27268.

Rai, V., U. Iyer, and U. V. Mani. "Effect of Tulasi (*Ocimum sanctum*) Leaf Powder Supplementation on Blood Sugar Levels, Serum Lipids, and Tissue Lipids in Diabetic Rats." *Plant Foods for Human Nutrition (Dordrecht, Netherlands)* 50, no. 1 (1997): 9–16. doi:10.1007/BF02436038.

Ramazanov, Zakir. "*Rhaponticum carthamoides*: Anabolic Effect of Whole Extract Is Superior to Individual Ecdysterones." In *Treasures of Siberian Phytomedicines:* Rhaponticum carthamoides. 2003.

Rea, Irene Maeve, David S. Gibson, Victoria McGilligan, Susan E. McNerlan, H. Denis Alexander, and Owen A. Ross. "Age and Age-Related Diseases: Role of Inflammation Triggers and Cytokines." *Frontiers in Immunology* 9 (April 2018): 586. doi:10.3389/fimmu.2018.00586.

Saeedi, M., K. Morteza-Semnani, and M.-R. Ghoreishi. "The Treatment of Atopic Dermatitis with Licorice Gel." *The Journal of Dermatological Treatment* 14, no. 3 (September 2003): 153–157. doi:10.1080/09546630310014369.

Sharma, Komal, and Maheep Bhatnagar. "*Asparagus racemosus* (Shatavari): A Versatile Female Tonic." *International Journal of Pharmaceutical & Biological Archives* 2, no. 3 (2011): 855–863.

Sharma, S., S. Ramji, S. Kumari, and J. S. Bapna. "Randomized Controlled Trial of *Asparagus racemosus* (Shatavari) as a Lactogogue in Lactational Inadequacy." *Indian Pediatrics* 33, no. 8 (August 1996): 675–677.

Singh, Narendra, Mohit Bhalla, Prashanti de Jager, and Marilena Gilca. "An Overview on Ashwagandha: A Rasayana (Rejuvenator) of Ayurveda." *African Journal of Traditional, Complementary, and Alternative Medicines* 8, no. 5 (2011): S208–S213. doi:10.4314/ajtcam.v8i5S.9.

Spasov, A. A., G. K. Wikman, V. B. Mandrikov, I. A. Mironova, and V. V. Neumoin. "A Double-Blind, Placebo-Controlled Pilot Study of the Stimulating and Adaptogenic Effect of *Rhodiola rosea* SHR-5 Extract on the Fatigue of Students Caused by Stress during an Examination Period with a Repeated Low-Dose Regimen." *Phytomedicine: International Journal of Phytotherapy and Phytopharmacology* 7, no. 2 (April 2000): 85–89.

Stancheva, S. L., and A. Mosharrof. "Effect of the Extract of *Rhodiola rosea* L. on the Content of the Brain Biogenic Monamines." *Medical Physiology: Proceedings of the Bulgarian Academy of Sciences* 40, no. 6 (1987): 85–87.

Stone, Mark, Alvin Ibarra, Mark Roller, Andrea Zangara, and Emma Stevenson. "A Pilot Investigation into the Effect of Maca Supplementation on Physical Activity and Sexual Desire in Sportsmen." *Journal of Ethnopharmacology. U.S. National Library of Medicine.* Accessed October 19, 2020. Pubmed.ncbi.nlm.nih.gov/19781622/.

Takada, Mitsutaka, Mai Fujimoto, and Kouichi Hosomi. "Association between Benzodiazepine Use and Dementia: Data Mining of Different Medical Databases." *International Journal of Medical Sciences* 13, no. 11 (October 2016): 825–834. doi:10.7150/ijms.16185.

Tiwari, Nimisha, Vivek Kumar Gupta, Pallavi Pandey, Dinesh Kumar Patel, Suchitra Banerjee, Mahendra Pandurang Darokar, and Anirban Pal. "Adjuvant Effect of *Asparagus racemosus* Willd. Derived Saponins in Antibody Production, Allergic Response and Pro-Inflammatory Cytokine Modulation." *Biomedicine & Pharmacotherapy* 86 (February 2017): 555–561. doi:10.1016/j.biopha.2016.11.087.

Trivedi, N. A., B. Mazumdar, J. D. Bhatt, and K. G. Hemavathi. "Effect of Shilajit on Blood Glucose and Lipid Profile in Alloxan-Induced Diabetic Rats." *Indian Journal of Pharmacology* 36, no. 6 (December 2004): 373–376.

Ven Murthy, Prabhakar K. Ranjekar, Charles Ramassamy, and Manasi Deshpande. "Scientific Basis for the Use of Indian Ayurvedic Medicinal Plants in the Treatment of Neurodegenerative Disorders: Ashwagandha." *Central Nervous System Agents in Medicinal Chemistry* 10, no. 3 (September 2010): 238–246. doi:10.2174 /1871524911006030238.

Verret, Claudia, Marie-Claude Guay, Claude Berthiaume, Phillip Gardiner, and Louise Béliveau. "A Physical Activity Program Improves Behavior and Cognitive Functions in Children with ADHD: An Exploratory Study." *Journal of Attention Disorders* 16, no. 1 (January 2012): 71–80. doi:10.1177/1087054710379735.

Wagner, H., H. Nörr, and H. Winterhoff. "Plant Adaptogens." *Phytomedicine: International Journal of Phytotherapy and Phytopharmacology* 1, no. 1 (June 1994): 63–76. doi:10.1016/S0944-7113(11)80025-5.

Wang, Ben-Xiang, Qiu-Li Zhou, Ming Yang, Yan Wang, Zhi-Yong Cui, Yong-Qiang Liu, and Takashi Ikejima. "Hypoglycemic Mechanism of Ginseng Glycopeptide." *Acta Pharmacologica Sinica* 24, no. 1 (January 2003): 61–66.

Wang, Chun-Mei, Rong-Shuang Yuan, Wen-Yue Zhuang, Jing-Hui Sun, Jin-Ying Wu, He Li, and Jian-Guang Chen. "*Schisandra* Polysaccharide Inhibits Hepatic Lipid Accumulation by Downregulating Expression of SREBPs in NAFLD Mice." *Lipids in Health and Disease* 15 (2016): 195. doi:10.1186/s12944-016-0358-5.

Wilson, Harold T. H., and John H. Edwards. "A Comparison of Glycyrrhetinic Acid and Hydrocortisone Ointments." *British Journal of Dermatology* 70, no. 12 (December 1958): 452–457. doi:10.1111/j.1365-2133.1958.tb13285.x.

Winters, Marie. "Ancient Medicine, Modern Use: *Withania somnifera* and Its Potential Role in Integrative Oncology." *Alternative Medicine Review* 11, no. 4 (December 2006): 269–277.

"*Withania somnifera* Monograph." *Alternative Medicine Review* 4, no. 2 (2004): 211–214.

Xia, Nan, Jie Li, Hongwei Wang, Jian Wang, and Yangtian Wang. "*Schisandra chinensis* and *Rhodiola rosea* Exert an Anti-Stress Effect on the HPA Axis and Reduce Hypothalamic c-Fos Expression in Rats Subjected to Repeated Stress." *Experimental and Therapeutic Medicine* 11, no. 1 (January 2016): 353–359. doi:10.3892/etm.2015.2882.

Zhang, Yu, Yu-Ting Wu, Wei Zheng, Xiao-Xuan Han, Yao-Huang Jiang, Pei-Lin Hu, Zhen-Xing Tang, and Lu-E Shi. "The Antibacterial Activity and Antibacterial Mechanism of a Polysaccharide from *Cordyceps cicadae*." *Journal of Functional Foods* 38 (November 2017): 273–279.

Zhou, L., W. Yang, Y. Xu, Q. Zhu, Z. Ma, T. Zhu, X. Ge, and J. Gao. "Short-Term Curative Effect of Cultured *Cordyceps sinensis* (Berk.) Sacc. Mycelia in Chronic Hepatitis B." *China Journal of Chinese Materia Medica* 15, no. 1 (January 1990): 53–65.

Index

Acknowledgments

I would like to acknowledge Southwest College of Naturopathic Medicine (SCNM) for providing me with an excellent and invaluable education. I would like to give an extra-special thanks to Dr. Patricia Gaines, ND, RH (AHG), Chair of the Botanical Medicine Department at SCNM. She was a wonderful mentor in both botanical and naturopathic medicine, and her passion for and guidance in the use of botanicals played an integral role in my education. I would also like to thank Gaia Herbs and Wise Woman Botanicals for providing me with invaluable opportunities to visit their facilities when I was a medical student and resident physician. Those experiences led to my awareness of and respect for how much love, intention, work, and quality control goes into manufacturing botanical products. I would also like to acknowledge the Southwest Conference on Botanical Medicine for continuing to provide exceptional opportunities to learn from many of the best herbalists in the field. All of these opportunities have led to my expertise in and love and passion for herbal medicine. Lastly, I would like to thank the amazing staff and editors at Callisto Media for making this book possible.

About the Author

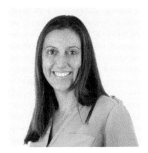

DR. RACHEL ROZELLE is a naturopathic physician currently practicing at the Windhorse Naturopathic Clinic in Brattleboro, Vermont. She completed medical school at Southwest College of Naturopathic Medicine in Tempe, Arizona, in 2012. Following a residency program in family medicine at Southwest Naturopathic Medical Center, she built a successful private practice in Santa Cruz, California. She then relocated to San Diego in order to expand her practice and join the faculty at Bastyr University in San Diego as an adjunct clinical provider. These experiences allowed her to hone her skills in pediatric and family medicine with an expertise in homeopathy and botanical medicine. She has served as a Board Member and Chair of the Professional Development Committee of the California Naturopathic Doctors Association. Recently, she had the honor of speaking at the international Joint American Homeopathic Conference on the topic of "Treating Mental and Emotional Pain in Children and Adolescents." Dr. Rozelle enjoys playing soccer, hiking, camping, teaching, helping others, and spending quality time with her family and friends.

Printed in the USA
CPSIA information can be obtained
at www.ICGtesting.com
LVHW072118110923
757457LV00004B/35

9 781647 399030